Emergencies Around Childbirth

Emergencies Around Childbirth

A HANDBOOK FOR MIDWIVES

Second Edition

Edited by

MAUREEN BOYLE
Senior Lecturer (Midwifery)
Thames Valley University
London

Radcliffe Publishing
London • New York

Radcliffe Publishing Ltd
33–41 Dallington Street
London
EC1V 0BB
United Kingdom

www.radcliffepublishing.com

Electronic catalogue and worldwide online ordering facility.

Every effort has been made to ensure the accuracy of these guidelines, and that the best information available has been used. This does not diminish the requirement to exercise clinical judgement, and neither the publisher nor the authors can accept any responsibility for their use in practice.

British Library Cataloguing in Publication Data

A catalogue record for this book is available from the British Library.

ISBN-13: 978 184619 336 1

The paper used for the text pages of this book is FSC® certified. FSC (The Forest Stewardship Council®) is an international network to promote responsible management of the world's forests.

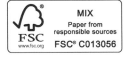

Typeset by Pindar NZ, Auckland, New Zealand
Printed and bound by TJI Digital, Padstow, Cornwall, UK

Contents

List of contributors

Judy Bothamley MA, PGCEA, ADM, RM, RGN
Senior Lecturer (Midwifery)
Thames Valley University
London

Maureen Boyle MSc, PGCEA, ADM, RM, RGN
Senior Lecturer (Midwifery)
Thames Valley University
London
Midwife, St Mary's Hospital
Imperial NHS Health Care
London

Helen Crafter MSc, PGCEA, ADM, RM, RGN, FP Cert
Senior Lecturer (Midwifery)
Thames Valley University
London

Elisabeth Hallewell MSc, BA(Hons), PGCEA, ADM, RM, RGN
Principal Lecturer (Midwifery)
Thames Valley University
London
Midwife, Ealing Hospital NHS Trust

Sandra McDonald MSc, PGCEA, ADM, RM, RGN
Senior Lecturer (Midwifery)
Thames Valley University
London

Judith Robbins BSc(Hons), RM, RGN
Clinical Placement Facilitator
St Mary's Hospital
Imperial NHS Health Care
London

Caroline Squire MSc, PGCEA, ADM, RM, RN, Lic Ac, Lic OHM
Senior Lecturer (Midwifery)
Thames Valley University
London

Hazel Sundle RM, RGN, Dip HE
Community Midwife
North Tyneside

Margaret Yerby MSc, PGCEA, ADM, RM, RGN
Senior Lecturer (Midwifery) (Retired)
Thames Valley University
London

CHAPTER 1

Introduction and professional issues

Maureen Boyle

As midwives we know that, usually, pregnancy and birth are normal physiological events. However, it is because this is our experience and because most common complications, such as postpartum haemorrhages, are easily dealt with that many midwives feel less than confident in uncommon or severe life-threatening emergency situations.

This book is intended to provide an easy-to access resource for practising midwives to enable them to build on their existing understanding of urgent or emergency situations. This second edition has built on the feedback from practising midwives, expanding what was considered especially useful and informative. In addition, there has also been an extra chapter (Chapter 13) added – in present-day midwifery practice, the psychosocial elements of our care are of increasing importance. Of course, during a life-threatening emergency, physical care rightly takes priority, but small actions which do not detract from this essential care may prevent lifelong psychological morbidity.

It has been identified that a knowledge of critical obstetric problems should be a high priority for obstetricians and that an understanding of the pathophysiology of various conditions and a knowledge of life-saving measures are integral to the effectiveness of treatment.[1] The same must be the case for midwives, who often have sole responsibility for the care of pregnant women and may be without immediate hospital and medical backup when an emergency happens.

The importance of extensive knowledge and expertise in high-risk situations goes beyond saving lives in an emergency, important as this is. If adverse events can be predicted and action taken to prevent them, or midwives are ready to deal with them effectively, the likelihood of improving outcomes for mothers and babies is increased. This does not mean that midwives should adopt the medical model of care,[2] but be more concerned with maintaining a wide-ranging and up-to-date knowledge base to ensure normality is maintained as far as possible. If a midwife has considered and reflected on all possible scenarios, including interventions which are appropriate while awaiting assistance, before they arise, she is likely

1

to increase the effectiveness of her actions and her confidence.

At first glance, it may be thought that a book about emergencies and high-risk situations around childbirth would give an underlying message that birth is not safe and that the authors would always advocate hospital birth in fully equipped centres. This is not the intended message. On the contrary, it is hoped that by encouraging midwives to enhance their confidence, knowledge and skills to deal with emergencies, a fear of complications would not be a barrier to offering home birth to women. Although this book deals with emergencies which are usually predicted and mean hospitalisation, all events discussed can occur unheralded. It is therefore important that midwives can deal effectively with urgent or emergency situations in the community, and for this reason 'first aid' actions are discussed in each chapter.

The need to screen women carefully before advising a home birth has been extensively explored,[3] although the dangers of hospital birth have been less well discussed. Hospital care and the growing number of interventions available may expose healthy women to more risks. In particular emergency caesarean sections may increase the chance of severe obstetric morbidity.[4,5]

Home births may do much to optimise women's physical and psychological experience of birth, so the slowly increasing trend of home births and the development of birthing centres should be encouraged. A barrier to this trend may be that most recently qualified midwives have never attended a home birth, and this may explain why there is evidence that midwives are not always willing to offer home births to women or do not feel confident in truly autonomous practice.[6–8] For example, many midwives fear maternal collapse whether it is as a result of an easily diagnosed cause such as haemorrhage or of an unknown cause, especially when attending a home birth or in other isolated circumstances.

It is important that midwives feel confident in their knowledge and do not bring anxieties and fears into the birthing environment.[9] Labouring women need to believe in their carers' abilities in order to be relaxed.[10] A good level of knowledge of high-risk conditions is mandatory if midwives are to gain and keep women's confidence. The published letter of a pregnant woman describing how an experienced midwife had asked her, 'What is HELLP syndrome?',[11] and a newspaper story of a woman dying following a home birth after a 'midwife had [a] crisis of confidence',[7] do nothing to encourage the readers' faith in the midwifery profession.

There is also a case for informed midwifery care, not only in emergency situations, but also when diagnosed obstetric complications have the potential for disaster. Although the obstetrician or other doctor will be the lead professional in such situations, ongoing midwifery care may have beneficial effects on the birth experience, making it seem as normal as possible by providing a focus on pregnancy and impending motherhood rather than on the pathology.[12]

It is most midwives' experience that labour interventions, including unplanned caesarean sections, are becoming more common. It is therefore likely that more women are experiencing physically and/or psychologically traumatic events around the time of birth.

One study showed an incidence of 12 cases of severe maternal morbidity for every 1000 deliveries.[4] These potentially life-threatening events may result in long-term physical effects. In more cases women may suffer psychological trauma which can lead to decisions to avoid further pregnancies or the symptoms of post-traumatic stress disorder. Situations where women experience powerlessness and lack of control are commonly accepted as a forerunner to psychological trauma (*see* Chapter 13). Debriefing after the birth is increasingly thought to be important and many midwives feel a postnatal discussion is a vital part of their after-care. Therefore, in many chapters medical interventions not in the midwife's realm have been included, as a review of these procedures may be useful if a midwife needs to discuss these processes with the woman postnatally. No matter how relieved or grateful a woman may feel after an emergency situation, it is very likely that her psychological health would be improved by being able to make sense of the situation through talking with a knowledgeable midwife.[13]

The *Report on Confidential Enquiries into Maternal Deaths*[14] makes sobering reading and is a useful resource for midwives, especially now they are more fully acknowledged as autonomous care providers. This document is an important source of information and midwives can learn lessons from others' actions in high-risk situations. The latest edition contains a chapter on midwifery practice and, among other issues, discusses midwifery accountability and advocacy, stating that they have a responsibility to challenge medical decisions when they believe that to be in the interests of the women in their care. However, to do this effectively, the midwife must have up-to-date medical knowledge. This book contains much

information that will hopefully enable midwives to enhance their understanding of high-risk medical/obstetrical situations that occur only infrequently. Although maternal mortality in the UK is now statistically low, the number of deaths where substandard care is implicated is too high for any complacency in those who care for women during childbirth.

An important part of midwifery care is attention to professional responsibilities, and many of these are directly impacted by emergency/high-risk care. Areas from the chapter on risk management (written by Carol Bates) in the first edition of this book are incorporated below, together with other relevant, and more recent, issues.

Risk management

Historically, childbirth was associated with risk and with good reason. Until the turn of the 20th century, maternal and perinatal mortality and morbidity rates in the Western world were high. During the 1920s, the maternal mortality rate was 4.4 deaths per 1000 total births, i.e. 3000 mothers died each year in England and Wales.[15] Women then had frequent pregnancies, often in very poor conditions.[16] Once social conditions improved and the importance of hygiene and nutrition was recognised, childbirth improved for both mother and baby. A risk management approach to pregnancy and childbirth has prevailed in Western society for a number of decades. This was a direct result of the obstetric view that pregnancy and birth could only be considered normal in retrospect. The World Health Organization (WHO)[17] considers that this risk approach to care has not been entirely effective because women considered to be low risk have unexpected complications and women considered to be high risk will go on to have an uneventful pregnancy and birth. It has also resulted in a disproportionately high number of women finding themselves in a high-risk category.

During the last three decades many risk-scoring systems have been developed. Their purpose is to classify individual women into defined categories for which action can then be planned. The problem with such a scoring system is that it clearly categorises women into high, intermediate and negligible risk and this will affect the care they receive. Enkin et al.[18] consider risk-scoring systems should be regarded with caution. They point out that while scoring can help to provide a minimum level of care in adequate settings, where provisions are inadequate they can result in a variety of unwarranted interventions and create unnecessary stress and anxiety for women. The WHO[17] considers that the foundation for good decision making is ongoing assessment of a woman's needs which can change, alongside an ongoing assessment of her birthing potential throughout pregnancy and labour, which can also change.

The increasing complexity of the risk approach to childbearing has had considerable impact upon midwifery practice. It has blurred the boundaries of normality in midwifery practice and while the midwife supports women in pregnancy and childbirth regardless of complications developing, a fundamental issue for midwives is the professional autonomy associated with normal birth. Gould[19] argued that midwives have failed to define normality because doctors have so closely defined abnormality and this has allowed the ensuing increasing medicalisation of what should be a normal physiological process for the majority of women.

As part of an effective risk management strategy, midwives should ensure that they have the skills required to attend a home birth. They need expert clinical skills in relation to the diagnosis of the onset of labour and monitoring the progress of labour. They should also be trained and competent in maternal and neonatal resuscitation. Midwives should carry the equipment that enables them to do this effectively (see Chapter 2). Midwives should also be aware of what emergency services are available, any guidelines or protocols related to calling them and the average transfer time to hospital.

The concept that each midwife is responsible and accountable for her own practice[20] has encouraged an individualised approach to risk management through the supervision of midwives rather than a more systematic approach. This approach has its drawbacks in that individual midwives may feel they are being targeted, which can lead to a climate of fear that is not helpful to effective clinical risk assessment and management.

A more systematic approach to risk management has been primarily obstetric led and this has resulted in some maternity units becoming permeated with an interventionist approach to care in the name of risk management. This process has to some extent marginalised midwifery practice and resulted in routine practices, many of which are not evidence-based (for example, a time limit on the duration of the second stage of labour), which have not been in the best interests of either women or the midwifery profession.

The success or otherwise of midwifery clinical risk assessment and management will depend to a large extent upon the clinical environment in which midwives work. Kirkham[21] conducted a study of the culture of midwifery in the National Health Service (NHS) in England and her findings reveal that the traditional midwifery activities of support and care continue but within organisations with very different values. Kirkham describes the voice of midwifery as being muted and midwives as being in a 'professional state of learned helplessness and guilt'.

Quilliam[22] suggests that while the modern discourse of risk management may be unfamiliar to midwives, the concept is not. She argues that midwives have always been taught to recognise abnormalities that require referral and are able to deal with life-threatening emergencies that require taking decisive action. Quilliam does not support the obstetric view that pregnancy can only be normal in retrospect, but she points out that if midwives actively embrace clinical risk management they will ensure that maternity services are both safe and woman-centred.

The Clinical Negligence Scheme for Trusts (CNST) was established by the NHS Executives in 1994 to enable trusts to fund the cost of clinical negligence litigation and to encourage and support effective management of risk and claims.[23] It is important for midwives to ensure they are kept up to date on maternity clinical risk management standards.[24] All trusts will have guidelines on what to do when an adverse incident occurs, and it is important midwives follow correct procedures to ensure the risk of a recurrence is minimised.[25] There have been many examples of both local and national audits that are based on individual incidents, but through critical incident audits, learning points and action plans can be identified.[26]

If midwives have a strong sense of professional identity, this will make the profession strong. Strong midwives are motivated to learn for enhanced competence and to become expert clinical practitioners, supporting and enhancing the physiological processes of childbearing, using interventions appropriately, able to manage abnormality and deal promptly and efficiently with emergencies. This is effective risk management.

Education

Except in an emergency, a practicing midwife shall not provide any care, or undertake any treatment, which she has not been trained to give. (Rule 6: NMC 2004)[20]

You must keep your knowledge and skills up to date throughout your working life.

You must take part in appropriate learning and practice activities that maintain and develop your competence and performance. (NMC 2008)[27]

As most emergencies are, thankfully, extremely rare events, it makes sense to undertake regular practice to ensure skills in these areas are not forgotten. Over the past few years, all maternity units have introduced regular mandatory 'skills drills' following the requirement from the Clinical Negligence Scheme for Trusts. For maximum effectiveness these should take place in the clinical area and involve the multidisciplinary team,[28] thus replicating a real emergency as closely as possible. *See* Chapter 9 for a discussion of the effectiveness of structured regular skills drills for shoulder dystocia – and this approach will of course be effective for all emergencies.

The *Seventh Annual Confidential Enquiry into Stillbirths and Deaths in Infancy*[29] identified a need for knowledgeable practitioners to deal with breech delivery at home, the majority of which will be unexpected. Since most breech presentations are now born by caesarean section midwives rarely experience vaginal breech births. There is therefore a clear need for midwives to regularly review this subject in particular to ensure their skills are up to date, especially if they lack practical experience.

Record keeping

A practising midwife shall keep, as contemporaneously as is reasonable, continuous and detailed records of observations made, care given and medicine and any form of pain relief administered by her to a woman or baby. (Rule 9: NMC 2004)[20]

Good record keeping is an integral part of nursing and midwifery practice, and is essential to the provision of safe and effective care. It is not an optional extra to be fitted in if circumstances allow. (NMC 2009)[30]

Guidelines on record keeping are published regularly by the Nursing and Midwifery Council (NMC) and it is a professional responsibility for the practising midwife to adhere to them. Many trusts are now introducing pro-formas for specific emergency situations (for example, shoulder dystocia). However, although this may enable times and actions to be more quickly and accurately identified, a pro-forma will never be as effective as notes, as inclusion of such aspects as communication with the woman/partner need to be documented. A study auditing records following cord prolapse[31] identified that the vast majority of women and their partners were not offered explanations following the event. Of course this may not be so, but professional record keeping considers that if the action was not documented it did not happen.

Griffith[32] suggests all records should be written with the knowledge that they may one day be scrutinised by a court as evidence. He suggests that the first impression the court has of a practitioner is the standard of the notes, and if they are not professional, it may be assumed that the care delivered was also not of a high standard. This is a salutary reminder, especially when the midwife may not feel like prioritising record keeping following a traumatic and exhausting emergency.

Supervision

The role of the Supervisor of Midwives initially centred on protecting the public by ensuring the standard of midwifery care was high. In fact Supervisors were known as 'Inspectors of Midwives' until 1937.[33] However, the role has expanded over the years and now involves a range of activities.[34] For the midwife involved in an emergency, who feels the need for support or debriefing, her Supervisor is certainly a person who should be able to undertake this.[35]

Conclusion

This book has been written by midwives for midwives, but the content is unsurprisingly very medically weighted.

Nevertheless, it is hoped by all the authors that this information will be used by midwives, not only to perhaps save lives and prevent morbidity, but also to enable women's experiences to become more fulfilling overall, as they are cared for by confident and knowledgeable midwives.

References

1 Van Geign H, Vothknecht S. (1996) Training in the management of critical problems: teacher's view. *Eur J Obstet Gynecol Reprod Biol.* **65**(1): 145–8.

2 Bryar R. (1995) *Theory for Midwifery Practice.* Basingstoke: Macmillan.

3 Campbell R. (1999) Review and assessment of selection criteria used when booking pregnant women at different places of birth. *Br J Obstet Gynaecol.* **106**(6): 550–6.

4 Waterstone M, Bewley S, Wolfe C. (2001) Incidence and predictors of severe obstetric morbidity: case-control study. *BMJ.* **322**: 1089–94.

5 Pallasmaa N, Ekblad U, Gissler M. (2008) Severe maternal morbidity and the mode of delivery. *Acta Obstet Gynecol Scand.* **87**(6): 662–8.

6 Magill-Cuerden J. (2001) A holiday in Devon: the RCM congress. *Br J Midwif.* **9**(6): 346–7.

7 Yeoman F. (2008) Joanne Whale died after home birth midwife had crisis of confidence. *The Times.* 15 May. Available at www.timesonline.co.uk/tol/news/uk/health/article3934513.ece

8 Vedam S, Stoll K, White S, *et al.* (2009) Nurse-midwives' experiences with planned home birth: impact on attitudes and practice. *Birth.* **36**(4): 274–82.

9 Weston R. (2001) When birth goes wrong. *Pract Midwife.* **4**(8): 10–12.

10 Green J, Curtis P, Price H, Renfrew M. (1998) *Continuing to Care.* Cheshire: Books for Midwives Press.

11 Thompson T. (1997) I knew more about HELLP than specialist midwife. *Action on Pre-eclampsia (APEC) Newsletter.* **14**: 7–8.

12 Lindsay P. (2006) Creating normality in a high-risk pregnancy. *Pract Midwife.* **9**(1): 16–19.

13 Axe S. (2000) Labour debriefing is crucial for good psychological care. *Br J Midwif.* **8**(10): 626–31.

14 Lewis G, editor. (2007) *The Confidential Enquiry into Maternal and Child Health (CEMACH). Saving Mothers' Lives: reviewing maternal deaths to make motherhood safer: 2003–2005. The Seventh Report on Confidential Enquiries into Maternal Deaths in the United Kingdom.* London: CEMACH.

15 The Royal College of Midwives. (2000) *Reassessing Risk: a midwifery perspective.* London: Royal College of Midwives.

16 Lewis J. (1990) Mothers and maternity policies in the 20th century. In: Garcia J, Kilpatrick R, Richards M, editors. *The Politics of Maternity Care.* Oxford: Clarendon Press. pp. 15–29.

17 World Health Organization. (1999) *Care in Normal Birth: a practical guide.* Geneva: World Health Organization.

18 Enkin M, Keirse M, Neilson, Crowther C, Duley L, Hodnett E, Hofmeyr J. (2000) *Guide to Effective Care in Pregnancy and Childbirth.* 3rd ed. Oxford: Oxford Medical Publications.

19 Gould D. (2000) Normal labour: a concept analysis. *J Adv Nurs.* **31**(2): 418–27.

20 Nursing and Midwifery Council (NMC). (2004) *Midwives Rules and Standards.* London: NMC.

21 Kirkham M. (1999) The culture of midwifery in the National Health Service in England. *J Adv Nurs.* **30**(3): 732–9.

22 Quilliam S. (1999) Clinical risk management in midwifery: what are midwives for? *MIDIRS Midwif Digest.* **9**(3): 280–4.

23 National Health Service Litigation Authority (NHSLA). (2005) *CNST, General Clinical Risk Management Standards.* London: NHSLA.

24 National Health Service Litigation Authority (NHSLA). (2009) *Clinical Negligence Scheme for Trusts Maternity Clinical Risk Management Standards.* Version 2.2009/10. London: NHS Litigation Authority.

25 Georgiou G. (2009) What do I do now? *RCM Midwives*. December/January: 42–3.

26 Brace V, Kernaghan D, Penney G. (2007) Learning from adverse clinical outcomes: major obstetric haemorrhage in Scotland, 2003–05. *BJOG*. **114**(11): 1388–96.

27 Nursing and Midwifery Council (NMC). (2008) *The Code: standards of conduct, performance and ethics for nurses and midwives*. London: NMC.

28 Rogers K. (2007) Skills drills training: the way forward. *RCM Midwives*. **10**(5): 218–19.

29 Maternal and Childbirth Research Consortium. (2000) *Confidential Enquiry into Stillbirth and Deaths in Infancy (Seventh Annual Report)*. London: CESDI.

30 Nursing and Midwifery Council (NMC). (2009) *Record Keeping: guidance for nurses and midwives*. London: NMC.

31 Rogers C, Schiavone N. (2008) Cord prolapse audit: recognition, management and outcome. *Br J Midwif*. **16**(5): 315–18.

32 Griffith R. (2007) Record keeping: midwives and the law. *Br J Midwif*. **15**(5): 303–4.

33 Mannion K. (2008) Statutory supervision of midwives. In: Peate I, Hamilton C, editors. *Becoming a Midwife in the 21st Century*. Chichester: John Wiley & Sons Ltd.

34 Burton S. (2008) 'Six hat supervision': a model for the supervisor of midwives. *Br J Midwif*. **16**(11): 736–42.

35 Kershaw K. (2007) Adverse clinical incidents: support for midwives. *RCM Midwives*. **10**(10): 462–5.

CHAPTER 2

Maternal and neonatal resuscitation

Maureen Boyle and Margaret Yerby

Maternal resuscitation

The necessity to resuscitate a pregnant woman or new mother is not a usual event. The occurrence of cardiac arrest in pregnancy and the puerperium has been estimated at around 1:30 000 deliveries,[1] but this number may well grow with the increasing numbers of older women, those with compromising lifestyles and those with pre-existing medical conditions, especially cardiac, becoming pregnant.[2]

Although some cardiac arrests can be anticipated, some are completely unexpected and all midwives are expected to be able to carry out basic life support, and assist with advanced life support. It is salutatory to note the Confidential Enquiry into Maternal and Child Health (CEMACH)[3] mentioned that resuscitation skills were poor in a number of the deaths they described. To enable acquisition and maintenance of proficiency in this skill, professional midwifery responsibilities include:

- arranging and/or attending regular updates and drills for resuscitation skills

- ensuring good working knowledge of equipment on an 'arrest trolley' including defibrillation and drugs
- working with representatives of the multidisciplinary team to review and revise equipment and drugs for use in a cardiac arrest
- ensuring all arrest trolleys (including drugs) are regularly checked and within date.

(*See* Boxes 2.4 and 2.5 for detail on typical resuscitation equipment.)

The most common causes of cardiopulmonary arrest are eclampsia (*see* Chapter 4) and hypovolaemia.[4] Hypovolaemia is caused through excessive blood loss at delivery or afterwards (*see* Chapter 10) or indeed at any time in pregnancy (*see* Chapter 5), creating an imbalance in the circulatory system. Some other less usual causes are also discussed in Chapter 12. Along with effective resuscitation is the need to establish what caused the arrest, and treatment of that is also necessary. The Resuscitation Council (UK)[5] has suggested that causes of cardiac arrest can be identified as fitting into eight categories, known as the 4Hs and the 4Ts. These are listed in Box 2.1, together with some of the more common obstetric reasons. Recognising complications of pregnancy that place women at risk can help clinicians in anticipating collapse in some circumstances.

> **BOX 2.1** Reversible causes for cardiac arrest: 4Hs & 4Ts (adapted from Adult Advanced Life Support Resuscitation Guidelines 2005)[5]
> - **H**ypoxia: eclampsia/cardiac conditions/status epilepticus/ severe asthma and other respiratory conditions/high spinal block/ Mendelson's syndrome
> - **H**ypovolaemia: haemorrhage (antenatal, intrapartum or postnatal)/ disseminated intravascular coagulation (DIC)
> - **H**ypo/hyperkalaemia/metabolic: renal failure
> - **H**ypothermia
> - **T**ension pneumothorax: severe asthma/trauma/complication of inserting central venous pressure (CVP) line
> - **T**amponade, cardiac: trauma
> - **T**oxins: magnesium sulphate toxicity/ septic shock/anaphylaxis
> - **T**hrombosis: amniotic fluid embolism/ pulmonary embolism.

If a woman collapses and is in a shocked state, evaluation of all the body systems has to be made in order to decide the way forward, as resuscitative measures may have to be taken. Box 2.2 lists the principles of care when this emergency takes place.

> **BOX 2.2** Principles of care following collapse
> - Early identification of the problems
> - **Call for help**
> - Maintenance of oxygen levels
> - Maintenance of circulation
> - Maintenance of fluid levels
> - Prevention of multiple organ failure
> - Evaluation of fetal condition.

Physiological events leading up to and following arrest

Collapse of the woman may be instantaneous or present initially as a condition of shock. She may exhibit a rapid but thready pulse, low blood pressure and pale sweaty skin. Consciousness may be impaired or she may seem disorientated or be exhibiting inappropriate behaviour – signs of hypoxia. Gasping respirations may be present, but are ineffective.[6] Total collapse may then occur. The heart will stop beating, respiration will cease and unless resuscitation takes place rapidly irreversible damage will take place. For survival, oxygen entry to the lung is required while the pumping action of the heart needs to be sustained to maintain blood circulation around the body and delivery of oxygen to the tissues in the body. It is imperative to maintain the woman's vital body systems.

Adaptive changes in physiology in pregnancy

The adaptation of maternal systems in pregnancy will alter the response of the mother to collapse.[1] For example, in severe blood loss the maternal blood pressure and pulse respond more slowly to a circulatory insult. By the time the maternal systems show the traditional responses to hypovolaemia (tachycardia and low blood pressure) the woman will be in a severe crisis and may need more intensive therapy to survive.[7]

Cardiac output increases in the first four weeks of pregnancy, which in turn increases the pulse rate. This is in response to an increase in blood volume, which is caused mainly by an increase in plasma volume. The blood supply to the uterus increases from 60 ml per minute to approximately 600 ml per minute at term. The increase in blood volume affects atrial naturetic peptide (ANP) because the heart senses the greater volume with stretch receptors, which increase ANP. ANP encourages more excretion of fluid from the kidneys and acts as a diuretic.[8] These physiological changes may mask the effect of shock in the pregnant woman. Therefore it is important to consider replacing fluid early on and to be prepared for collapse, rather than to wait for the normal signs and symptoms of hypovolaemia in the pregnant woman. Fluid balance can be a challenge when treating pregnant women – if a woman has suffered trauma, for example, rapid fluid replacement may be necessary; however, the dangers of fluid overload must never be forgotten.

Physiological changes when body systems are not sustained

When the heart stops beating circulation of blood stops, all the cells in the body become hypoxic and cell metabolism alters to create an acidosis. Blood pH should be maintained at between 7.35 and 7.45. At cellular level, metabolism requires oxygen to produce adenosine triphosphate (ATP), the energy source to power the cells' functions, the end products being carbon dioxide and water.

Carbon dioxide is normally a respiratory stimulant, but a build-up of it in a situation where a woman has collapsed is detrimental to the balance of body fluids. Without constant delivery of fluid via the circulatory system cellular function becomes anaerobic and causes acidosis. The respiratory system fails, the blood does not get supplied with oxygen, and carbon dioxide builds up in the capillary beds and is not excreted. The kidneys are no longer supplied with filtrate or oxygen to assist them to break down excess substrates in the blood, maintain a balance and excrete harmful substances. The brain is unable to function without oxygen and cell death quickly occurs.

The arterial base deficit measurement of blood depicts the available buffering solutions in the blood that could correct the acid–base balance physiologically (the normal range being between –2 to +2 mmol/l). Lactate levels measure acidosis and normally are <2.5 mmol/l of blood. These measurements are easily tested in the laboratory, but lactate levels may alter in relation to liver damage or sepsis, as clearance is not so efficient.[9] Normal blood values are given in Box 2.3. It is important to consider that blood circulation and respiration must be maintained with an adequate circulating fluid volume for the body to survive cardiopulmonary collapse.[10]

BOX 2.3 Normal blood levels
- Lactate <2.5 mmol/l
- Base deficit –2 to +2 mmol/l
- pH 7.35–7.45
- pCO_2 35–45 mmHg
- pO_2 80–100 mmHg

In pregnancy postural hypotension is created when the woman is in the dorsal position for periods of time as the enlarging uterus presses on the inferior vena cava and descending aorta. It occurs from the second trimester onwards and as the fetus grows it becomes more of a problem. At term these blood vessels can be completely blocked when supine. This will result in a decrease in cardiac stroke volume of up to 70%.[11]

During pregnancy large amounts of blood pool in the peripheral circulation. If the woman is in labour and has epidural analgesia the situation will be exacerbated because the sympathetic nervous system has been paralysed to facilitate pain relief and thus venous return is impaired. Traditionally, resuscitation would be performed on a patient in the dorsal position. However, in the pregnant woman it is important to maintain venous return and good circulation, so the wedge position, which is a left lateral tilt, is used (*see* Figures 2.1 and 2.2). Alternatively (or additionally), the uterus can be manually displaced if there are sufficient helpers available.[6] Following trauma it is important to consider the possibility of neck injury and to immobilise the neck prior to tilting the pregnant woman.[12]

A key role of the midwife is early identification and intervention to prevent collapse if possible. Therefore, midwives must always be alert to warning signs, such as rapid thready pulse, altered consciousness, pallor, cyanosis or abnormal respirations (less than 10, more than 30 or gasping/laboured) to ensure an early referral is made.[13] Once an emergency requiring resuscitative measures has been identified, the maternal well-being takes precedence, for if maternal life support is achieved there is a good chance that the fetus will survive.

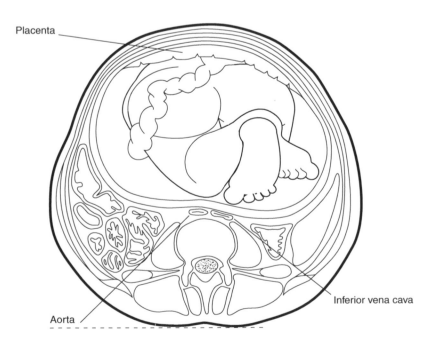

FIGURE 2.1 Aortal and inferior vena caval compression in dorsal position

BOX 2.4 Usual resuscitation equipment available in hospital

Equipment ready for use on top of trolley
- Portable oxygen and relevant masks
- Pocket masks
- Rebreathing unit (masks/bag)
- Electrocardiograph (ECG) pads to attach to patient
- Defibrillation pads and defibrillator
- Suction catheters.

Other equipment (in drawers)
- Endotracheal tubes (ET) in various sizes
- Airways
- Introducer for ET tubes, ET ties
- Scissors
- Intravenous equipment.

Cannulae, giving sets, intravenous fluids
- Dextrose 5%
- Sodium chloride 0.9%

- Gelofusine or other colloid
- Small ampoules of sodium chloride/ water for injection.

Drugs (in sealed, dated boxes)
- Atropine
- Adrenaline
- Adenosine
- Amiodarone
- Calcium chloride 10%
- Calcium gluconate
- Diazemuls
- Glucose 5%
- Lidocaine 2%
- Narcan® (naloxone)
- Sodium bicarbonate 8.4%
- Verapamil.

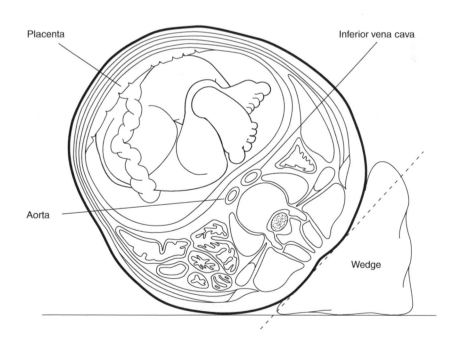

FIGURE 2.2 Left lateral tilt relieves compression

BOX 2.5 Resuscitation equipment available at home births
- Portable oxygen
- Face masks
- Ambubags
- Portable suction
- Cannulae and giving sets
- Intravenous fluids.

Principles of life support in pregnancy

Because the need for cardiopulmonary resuscitation is rare in pregnancy little has been written specifically on the support of women who collapse and require it. Guidelines must be taken from the principles of adult life support laid down by the Resuscitation Council (UK). In 2005 the Resuscitation Council (UK) issued new guidelines for basic adult resuscitation[14] with a view to simplifying – and therefore making more effective – several areas of basic resuscitation (*see* Figure 2.3).

In any life-threatening event it is important to remember that help is required. This can usually be obtained by ringing for an ambulance and paramedic assistance if the woman is outside the hospital or by activating the emergency bell in a hospital situation to summon other midwives who will then request the cardiac arrest team. In hospital it is also important to ensure the arrest team can access the maternity unit and know exactly where to come.[3] If the cardiac arrest occurs outside the hospital it is important to instruct someone to obtain help, or if alone phone before commencing resuscitation. It is imperative to obtain medical aid as soon as possible because outcomes are better if defibrillation occurs earlier rather than later.[14]

At the first signs of collapse a pregnant woman should be immediately turned to

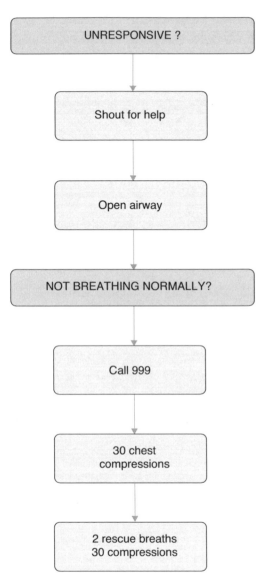

FIGURE 2.3 Adult basic life support (reproduced with the permission of the Resuscitation Council UK)

the left lateral position and firmly wedged at a left tilt using pillows or a foam wedge. As previously discussed (*see* Figures 2.1 and 2.2), this will aid venous return and prevent postural hypotension. If pillows or foam are not available an assistant can kneel behind the woman to act as a wedge and stabilise the left tilt position. It must be remembered that whatever support for the 'tilt' is used, it must provide a solid base or cardiac compressions will be ineffective. Evaluation can be done in the usual way: look, feel, listen for chest movement. The basic principles of ABC prevail for initial assessment:

A – airway
B – breathing
C – circulation.

Cardiopulmonary resuscitation (CPR)

A *precordial thump* may be given if the cardiac arrest is observed, but it needs to be undertaken immediately and only by healthcare professionals trained in the technique.[5]

The *airway* can be maintained by tilting the head, applying pressure on the forehead with one hand and lifting the chin up with the fingertips of the other hand, or performing a jaw thrust manoeuvre if the airway is still obstructed by finding the angle of the jaw with the fingers and pushing in an upward and forward movement. If the patient has sustained any trauma to the neck, care should be taken not to over-extend the neck until an X-ray has ruled out any neck problems.

After ensuring a clear airway, and observing a lack of respirations, basic resuscitation begins with *chest compressions* (*see* Figure 2.3 for the adult basic life support algorithm). Cardiac compression should be undertaken with the pregnant woman in the left tilt position, and in the knowledge that the heart is displaced to the left in pregnancy. To perform cardiac compression, place the heel

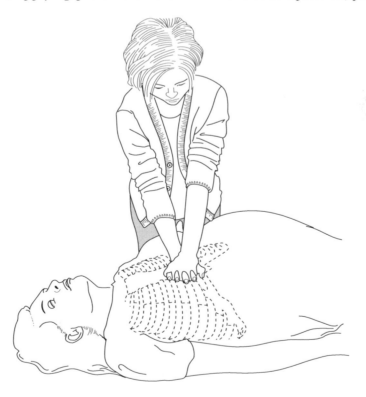

FIGURE 2.4 Hand position for chest compression

of one hand in the centre of the chest and place the heel of the other hand on top of the first, interlocking the fingers. Pressure should not be applied over the ribs or the bottom of the sternum/abdomen. Lock the hands together, straighten the arms and, placing weight on the hands from vertically above the woman, press down on the sternum for 30 compressions (*see* Figure 2.4). After every compression the hands should not be moved, but all pressure should be released. Repeat this action at a rate of about 100 times a minute, depressing the sternum 4–5 cm each time. Compression and release should take an equal amount of time.

After 30 compressions, check the airway is open again, and pinching the nose closed (*see* Figure 2.5) take a normal breath, and, sealing lips around the woman's mouth, blow steadily while also watching to ensure her chest rises. After removing your mouth (and her chest should fall as air is released), repeat this action. Then return to chest compressions. These actions should be continued at a ratio of 30 chest compressions to two rescue breaths until help arrives. Do not stop to check results of this CPR unless she begins to breathe normally. The UK Resuscitation Council[14] says that if the rescuer is unable or unwilling to give rescue breaths, chest compressions should be maintained at a rate of about 100 per minute.

If available, two people should give CPR at the same ratio of 30 chest compressions to two breaths until the arrest team arrives. It is important for the rescuers to change over about every two

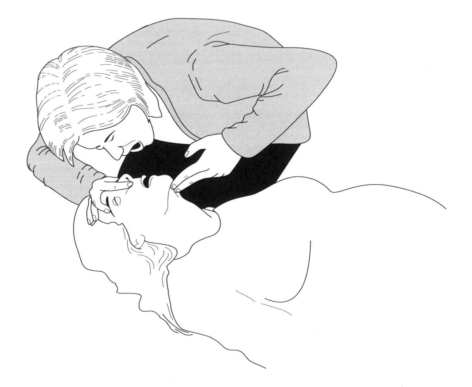

FIGURE 2.5 Head position for mouth-to-mouth ventilation

minutes to prevent fatigue when undertaking compressions, and this should be done with a minimum of delay to resuscitation. If the midwife has access to a bag-mask (ambubag) then breaths will be given at the same ratio (*see* Figure 2.6 for positioning).

To continue the resuscitation process after skilled help arrives (*see* Figure 2.7 for the adult advanced life support algorithm), the airway needs to be maintained and an endotracheal tube inserted. This could be difficult as changes in pregnancy can cause oedema of the neck tissues or the glottis and therefore enlargement of the neck. To prevent problems an experienced obstetric anaesthetist should insert the tube. Cricoid pressure during intubation will prevent the acid contents of the stomach, which may not be empty, from blocking the airway. CPR should be maintained at 30:2 until the airway is secured, then chest compressions should be continued with pausing.

Defibrillation

Once resuscitation has commenced the heart may be working erratically and defibrillation (a shock delivered to 'terminate fibrillation') to stabilise heart action might be required. If the ventricular pumping action is not stabilised, rescue attempts will not be successful as the pumping action of the heart is necessary not only for general circulation but also to supply oxygen to the myocardium of the heart.[15]

The use of defibrillation is dependent on the heart rhythm, and these are divided into two groups. Arrhythmias that can be shocked are ventricular fibrillation (VF)

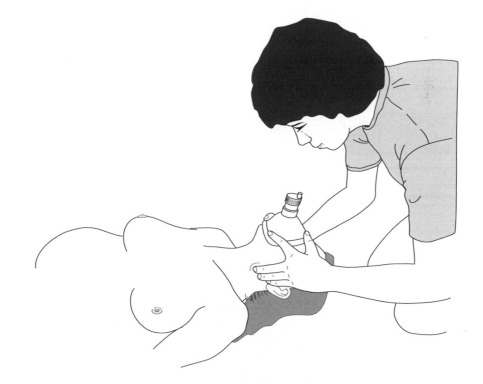

FIGURE 2.6 Head position for performing mouth-to-mask ventilation

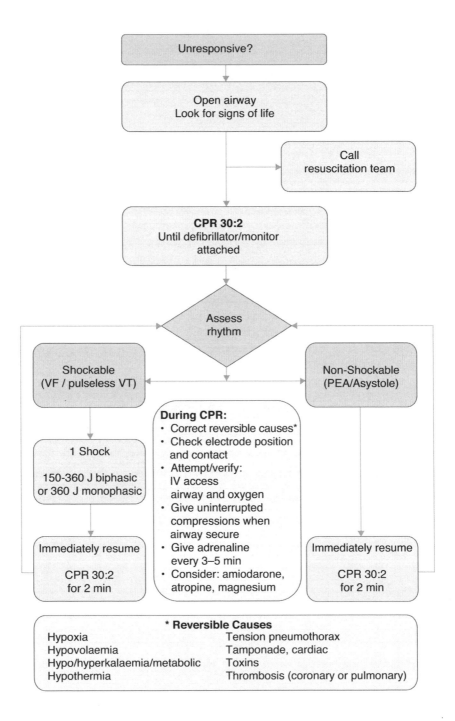

FIGURE 2.7 Adult advanced life support (reproduced with the permission of the Resuscitation Council UK)

and pulseless ventricular tachycardia (VT). VF/VT are less common in pregnancy as they are associated with ischaemic heart disease.[16] The arrhythmias where defibrillation is not effective are pulseless electrical activity (PEA) or asystole, and in these cases CPR (as described previously) at a rate of 30:2 should be continued. After the airway is secured, continuous compressions are maintained, ventilation is given at a rate of about 10/minute and drug treatment is used.

The heart rhythm can be identified via an ECG or automated defibrillator. If the heart rhythm is shockable, defibrillation will be carried out. Automated defibrillators (shock advisory defibrillators: AED), which are increasingly accessible, not only to first aiders in various workplaces but also in hospitals, analyse the rhythm of the heart, give voice prompts and also deliver an automatically measured current to the woman. Electrodes should be positioned on the sternum and to the left of the chest wall (midaxillary between the fifth and sixth ribs), and an electric shock is then passed through the heart. If a traditional machine is used, paddles are positioned identically to the electrodes for the automated defibrillator (*see* Figure 2.8).

It is important to ensure all personnel have no contact with the woman while she is being shocked, and this includes indirect contact, for example touching the bed. It is usual to call out 'ALL CLEAR' immediately prior to the shock, and this warning should be heeded. Because of the danger of fire, open sources of oxygen should also be temporarily removed.

CPR should immediately be resumed following the shock, and the resuscitation sequence (*see* Figure 2.7) should continue under the direction of the advanced life support professional (usually an anaesthetist in a hospital situation).

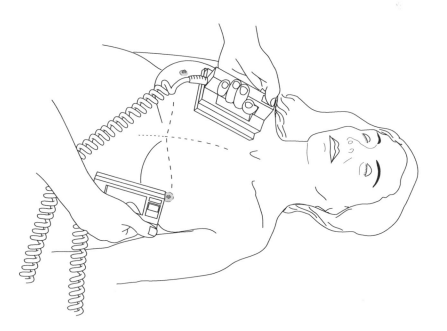

FIGURE 2.8 Chest and paddle positions for defibrillation

Fluid replacement

At the first signs of a woman's condition deteriorating measures should be taken to secure an IV access and to prevent it worsening by administering intravenous fluids. In a community setting the midwife could commence giving fluids intravenously if she has the equipment, but if not the paramedic will do so on arrival. When an arrest has taken place support of respiration and cardiac output (CPR) is undertaken. Once advanced life support is available (for example after arrival at the hospital, or after the arrest team has arrived) it is important to address the reason for the arrest. All causes (and management of the arrest itself) will need some form of intravenous drugs, and siting cannulae and administration of intravenous fluids is an essential component of this support. Inadequate perfusion creates a metabolic acidosis and if the base deficit and lactate are not stabilised adult respiratory distress syndrome (ARDS) may result. Women with an abnormal base deficit are more likely to suffer ARDS and its consequent multiple organ failure.

The aim of fluid replacement is to balance the chemical components of the blood and to maintain blood pressure if it is low. However, in itself, fluid infusion can be detrimental as it could alter the body's thermal balance and disturb blood clots. Crystalloids such as normal saline, 5% dextrose and dextrose saline have been shown to reduce blood viscosity, lower haematocrit and dilute clotting factors, so it is important to control haemorrhage prior to infusion with fluids.[17] The quicker normal blood patterns are stabilised, the better the outcome. It is important to maintain careful records of fluids used in an emergency situation, and be aware of the dangers of overloading the woman's system.

Drugs

Drugs are a vital part of resuscitation, and although they will be administered by the arrest team, the midwife needs to not only have a knowledge of how to obtain them quickly but also to anticipate what may be used. Note that all drugs given intravenously peripherally must be followed by at least 20 ml of flush. Box 2.6 describes the drugs commonly used in a cardiac arrest.

Caesarean section

Focus of care is always directed towards the woman; however, effective treatment of the woman will also treat the fetus. Resuscitation guidelines suggest that if resuscitation is still necessary after five minutes, a caesarean section should be carried out as delivery of the baby may benefit the mother. This will improve maternal cardiac output and stroke volume by some 30%, and enable better recovery. Resuscitation is more effective without the fetus *in utero*.[18]

Caesarean section should be carried out swiftly and efficiently once the decision has been made. It has been suggested that normal operating room routines only waste time, and initially only a scalpel is necessary.[19] CPR should be continued during the caesarean section.[19] The midwife should anticipate this action during any arrest of a pregnant woman, warning the arrest team when four minutes have passed, and ensuring equipment and paediatric support is ready. Although perinatal outcome is often poor following peri/post-mortem caesarean section, the number of babies surviving in these circumstances is increasing, but this is of

---

BOX 2.6 Drugs commonly used to support systems following the arrival of the multidisciplinary team

Adrenaline (epinephrine)
- Usually given alternatively with shocks, or regularly (every 3–5 minutes) if a non-shockable rhythm is present, intravenously or into the endotracheal tube.
- Adrenaline is a sympathomimetic drug that increases the heart rate and its force of contraction, which improves blood flow to the vital organs.
- It is the first medication to be administered in an arrest situation. However, its use in pregnancy does mean that blood is drawn away from the uterus, thus potentially affecting uteroplacental perfusion.

Amiodarone
- Amiodarone is an antiarrhythmic and has been shown to be effective in arrests outside hospital and also in situations when ventricular fibrillation or pulseless ventricular tachycardia has not been successfully treated with defibrillation.

Atropine
- Atropine blocks the action of the vagus nerve on the sinoatrial node and atrioventricular node, thus improving heart conduction in hypotension and bradycardia.

Lignocaine (lidocaine)
- Given intravenously, usually only when amiodarone is not available.
- Lignocaine stabilises ventricular fibrillation and prevents ectopic activity or extra beats in the ventricles.
- It is not effective in the management of atrial arrhythmias.
- Overdose of lignocaine causes drowsiness, confusion and muscular twitching, which can be quickly reversed by discontinuing the drug.

Calcium chloride
- For treatment of magnesium overdose, or hyperkalaemia.

Sodium bicarbonate
- Used during a cardiac arrest to treat acidosis.

---

course highly dependent on the gestation and where the delivery takes place.[3]

Support and outcomes

The first part of this chapter dealt with cardiac resuscitation of the pregnant woman, but little has been said regarding possible outcomes for the mother or the family. At best, resuscitation will be successful with full recovery of the mother and a healthy baby. At worst, the family may experience not only the loss of a loved one, but also the loss of the unborn baby. They may have observed the collapse and death, and the effect this may have on their grief process may be profound.

This subject is not easily researched or indeed written about. There is also little in the literature specific to maternal resuscitation in pregnancy and childbirth scenarios, with most reports from casualty or intensive care environments. However, when questioned, some relatives have said that they preferred to stay while resuscitation attempts were made, regardless of the consequences of the procedure, and it helped them to come to terms with the death of the loved one if that was the outcome. There is increasing evidence that shows both satisfaction and psychological benefit for relatives who observed resuscitation.[20] Support is all-important here and it is imperative that a member of staff is available to discuss and explain events, if possible while they are happening.[21,22]

A relevant report by a sister who witnessed her brother's accident and subsequent attempted resuscitation was published in the *British Medical Journal*.[23] She was very positive about the fact that she had been with her brother and stated that she had discussed the processes involved with doctors and nurses who were divided in their opinions as to the advantages and disadvantages of the observation of resuscitation procedures by relatives. Such involvement may help the grief process, but it may be difficult for health professionals to see the benefits at the time. Perhaps professionals need to discuss this subject openly and review policy on the involvement of relatives at resuscitation events.[24]

Midwives should also give support to each other as the necessity for resuscitation of a mother is such a rare and tragic occurrence that it is very distressing for all concerned. The Supervisor of Midwives would have a very important role to play in these circumstances.

Neonatal resuscitation

The birth of a baby always brings anticipation and a sense of achievement on completion, and it is expected that the baby will cry or gasp. This is the natural reflex for a baby entering the world as its chest walls, having been squeezed by the vagina, are suddenly released and lung expansion can take place. As the baby begins to breathe, oxygen permeates the cells and the skin colour rapidly changes from blue to pink.

On occasions and sometimes totally unexpectedly there is silence in the room as the baby is born. A baby with cyanosed skin may give a quiet gasp. If a good heartbeat can be felt or heard, circulation has been maintained, but there may still be no good cry or signs of respiration. This is a scenario every midwife will recognise and be prepared to manage with skill and competence.

The list of conditions which increase risk for the neonate is formidable (*see* Box 2.7) but gives the practitioner some guidance on when resuscitation of a neonate or transfer of a mother in labour to hospital may become necessary. All events, including conditions that increase risk, are required to be recorded in the mother's notes and it has been reported in many situations where a baby has died that such communication could have been important in the prevention of neonatal death.[25] However, it is salutary to note that it has been suggested that approximately 20% of babies that needed resuscitation did so unexpectedly, with no signs during pregnancy or labour.[26]

Therefore, it is vital that midwives keep up to date with neonatal resuscitation skills. This is also particularly important because 70% of all normal births are supervised by midwives and so they are often the first professional to diagnose collapse in the newborn and instigate resuscitation. It is also important that midwives should prioritise the checking of resuscitation equipment and drugs available during each labour they attend,

BOX 2.7 Conditions which increase risk for the neonate

Antepartum factors

- Maternal history of medical disease, e.g. diabetes, hypertension, heart disease
- Pre-eclampsia
- Anaemia or isoimmunisation
- Previous fetal or neonatal death
- Haemorrhage in the second or third trimesters
- Maternal infection
- Multiple pregnancy
- Maternal substance abuse, e.g. drugs, alcohol or smoking
- Fetal abnormality, including intrauterine growth restriction (IUGR)
- No antenatal care
- Age <16 or >35
- Increase or decrease in liquor volume
- Preterm or post-term gestation.

Intrapartum factors

- Abruptio placentae or placenta praevia
- Prolapsed cord
- Preterm labour
- Precipitous labour
- Prolonged labour >24 hours
- Prolonged rupture of membranes >18 hours
- Intrapartum maternal pyrexia
- Prolonged second stage of labour >2 hours
- Abnormal presentation or malposition of the fetus
- Abnormal uterine action, leading to uterine atony
- Meconium-stained liquor
- Narcotics administered to the mother within 3–4 hours of birth
- Abnormal heart rate patterns on cardiotocography (CTG)
- Forceps or ventouse extraction
- Emergency caesarean section and/or general anaesthesia.

to ensure effective resuscitation can be carried out if it is needed.

Intrapartum and the fetus

In utero, the fetus is protected by membranes and liquor; the placenta is its life support system. The fetus obtains oxygen from maternal oxygen supplies via the placenta and if these are inadequate at any time the heart rate patterns of the fetus change. The lungs, heart and some components of the blood of the fetus are adapted to survive in this enclosed environment (*see* Box 2.8).

There are three principal shunts (*see* Box 2.8) which facilitate a good supply of oxygen to the vital organs. When the blood enters the system from the placenta oxygenation is high, but it soon mixes with the blood already in circulation which has less oxygen. The shunts within the system ensure that the vital organs obtain higher levels of oxygen-saturated blood from the heart as quickly as possible.[27] As the fetus receives oxygen from the mother it also transfers excreted products to her. This momentarily alters pH values in the mother and permits greater levels of oxygen to diffuse across to the fetus (the Bohr effect).[10] In addition haemoglobin content is higher in fetal blood, which therefore attracts more oxygen.

As labour commences the delivery of oxygen to the fetus may be affected. Uterine contractions may affect the volume of blood circulating at placental level and/or the cord may become

---

BOX 2.8 Fetal adaptation *in utero*

Heart
- Ventricles pump in parallel.

Three principal shunts
- Ductus venosus: diverts highly oxygenated blood to the inferior vena cava.
- Foramen ovale: diverts highly oxygenated blood to the left side of the heart in order to supply the body.
- Ductus arteriosus: diverts blood away from the non-expanding lungs to the aorta.

Blood
- Higher haemoglobin levels, which have a higher binding capacity to oxygen because of its structure (fetal haemoglobin).

---

trapped between the pelvis and soft tissues during the descent of the fetus. The healthy fetus will automatically react to this disruption by an alteration in heart rate that is brought about by the baroreceptors in the aortic arch and carotid sinuses, which sense the partial pressure of oxygen dissolved in blood plasma. The chemoreceptors in the peripheral and brain systems are sensitive to blood pH levels.[10] A variable heart rate therefore indicates the fetus' ability to adapt to varying circumstances. A transitory rise in heart rate may indicate intrauterine asphyxia and would mean a degree of stress for the fetus. The mature fetus that is stressed will often pass meconium and this is brought about by the overproduction of motilin, a bowel hormone which increases gut motility in these circumstances. It is expected that the preterm fetus has a higher heart rate, which becomes more stable with maturity.

The level of acidosis is important when assessing fetal well-being in labour. Any Ph levels over 7.25 are normal, those between 7.20 and 7.25 are viewed as pre-acidotic and levels below 7.20 indicate acidosis. The level of acidosis indicates the level of lactic acid in the fetal systems, which rises due to lack of oxygen and an increase in carbon dioxide levels in the bloodstream. This indicates hypoxia *in utero*. The slow rise to the baseline rate following a bradycardial incident indicates the return of more adequate oxygen levels for the fetus.

All observations of the fetal condition by whatever means are important. Abnormal findings will alert the midwife to the fact that the fetus may require earlier rather than later delivery. However, there are some situations (*see* Box 2.9) in which the midwife will need to observe the fetus even more carefully in labour in anticipation of problems at birth. Fetal distress and/or meconium-stained liquor are warning signs in labour that would influence the midwife's decision to transfer the mother to hospital and to call for a paediatrician when birth is imminent.

At birth the transition to extrauterine life occurs almost instantly. The occlusion of the cord alters pressures in the right side of the heart and the infant's first breath fills the lungs with air.[28] If the baby does not take that first breath (*see* Box 2.9 for potential reasons for failure to do so) the midwife should instigate closer observation and ensure resuscitative measures are commenced promptly.

> **BOX 2.9** Reasons for failure of the newborn to commence respiration (adapted from Drew *et al.*[29])
> - Adverse intrapartum events, e.g. difficult labour, fetal distress
> - Drugs given to the mother
> - Immaturity
> - Sepsis
> - Abnormalities of the respiratory system, i.e. diaphragmatic hernia, obstruction
> - Trauma.

The Apgar score (*see* Table 2.1 for a typical example) is the traditional assessment of newborn well-being, and is still a valid tool.[30] It consists of a scoring system based on points out of 10, assessing heart rate, respiratory effort, muscle tone, reflex response and colour. It is a quick and easy assessment of the newborn's condition at birth made at one and five minutes (and at 10 minutes if necessary) and provides a guide to further development in the neonate's systems.[30] The reliability of the Apgar score versus readings of the pH of the umbilical arterial blood at birth in respect of success in predicting adverse neonatal outcomes has been questioned, but has been proved to be an appropriate assessment tool.[31]

It is important that the room in which the child will be born is prepared prior to birth. A warm atmosphere is essential and all relevant equipment should be checked and maintained, especially when a birth is expected. As soon as the birth has occurred, the baby should be dried and the midwife will observe the overall condition. In many circumstances the baby may be delivered into the mother's arms and then dried and maintained with skin-to-skin contact. If the baby does not show signs of respiratory effort and continues to remain cyanosed, the ABC of resuscitation should be followed (*see* Figure 2.9).

When cutting the cord of a baby that is in need of resuscitation, consideration should be made to keep a long length, as intra-umbilical catheterisation may be necessary. In the vast majority of cases, however, it is not, and the cord can then be trimmed to the normal length later. It is also worth noting that the cord site should be checked as resuscitation is being undertaken – it is not unknown for a clamp to be inadequately applied or slip, and the baby may lose a significant amount of blood, which will be hidden by blankets keeping him/her warm.

The Paediatric Working Group[32] suggest that 'approximately 5%–10% of newborns require some degree of active

TABLE 2.1 Apgar scoring system

	Score of 0	Score of 1	Score of 2
Respiratory effort	absent	Slow/irregular	good
Heart rate	absent	<100	≥100
Trunk colour	pale	blue	pink
Muscle tone	limp	flexion	active
Response to stimulation	absent	grimace	good

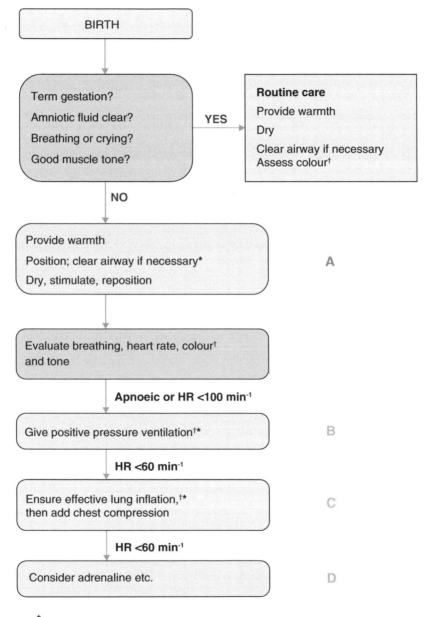

* Tracheal intubation may be considered at several steps
† Consider supplemental oxygen at any stage if cyanosis persists

FIGURE 2.9 Newborn life support (reproduced with the permission of the Resuscitation Council UK)

resuscitation at birth'. In a labour ward delivering 20 babies a day this would mean that two of those babies would require active resuscitation – a sobering thought and one that emphasises the necessity for every midwife to be competent in resuscitation skills.

Life support in the newborn
Warmth

It is vital to maintain the baby's temperature at a constant level, as a drop in temperature will mean that stored glucose will be used to produce more heat to raise the temperature and the neonate will require more oxygen to efficiently carry out cell metabolism.[10] Also, if a baby is allowed to become cold, this will inhibit its ability to produce surfactant.

Ventilation

A face mask with a pressure bag is the most common form of early ventilation once the airway is cleared[29] (*see* Figure 2.10). For some time it has not been evidence-based practice to suction a baby born in the presence of meconium 'on the perineum' (i.e. after the birth of the head

and before the birth of the shoulders).[33] Also, in the presence of meconium, it has been traditional to suction a baby under direct vision after endotracheal intubation to clear thick meconium from the vocal cords and prevent meconium aspiration syndrome. However, a recent Cochrane review has suggested that it is not necessary to intubate and suction the 'vigorous term infant' as there seem to be no benefits to outcomes over and above oropharyngeal suction.[34,35] However, the Resuscitation Council has advised in their guidelines for neonatal resuscitation[35] that if the baby is born through thick meconium and is unresponsive, the oropharynx should be cleared of meconium. It should be noted that vigorous pharyngeal suction should be avoided as it can cause a reflex apnoea.[26]

The baby's head should be positioned in 'neutral' to achieve the optimum airway opening (*see* Figure 2.11). If the baby is floppy, it may also be necessary to apply a chin lift or jaw thrust. If there are not adequate respirations after about 90 seconds, the baby should be given five inflation breaths. These breaths should be

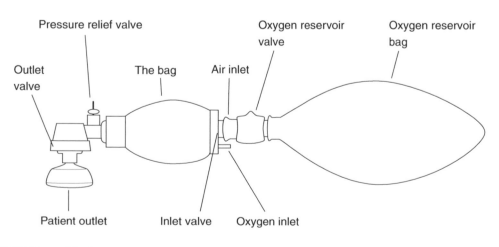

FIGURE 2.10 Mask

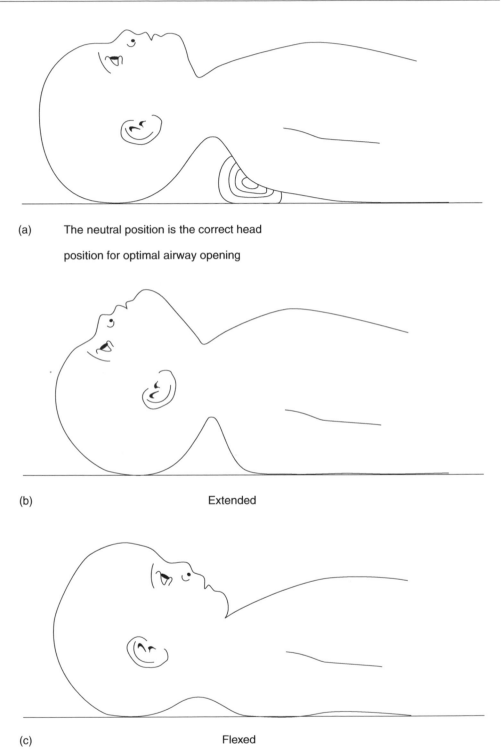

(a)   The neutral position is the correct head

position for optimal airway opening

(b)   Extended

(c)   Flexed

FIGURE 2.11 Head position for optimum airway opening

sustained for 2–3 seconds, and the baby's chest should be observed to ensure it rises with each breath.

Masks used for ventilation should fit the baby well by not occluding the eyes or overlapping the chin. If the mask does not fit correctly, oxygen pressure will not be maintained and delivery will be poor. An unimpeded airway should be maintained by a gentle/minimal lifting of the chin while maintaining a good fit with the mask.

When the heart rate is more than 100 beats per minute, ventilation can be stopped and the baby observed. If the baby continues to be slow to respire independently, and the heart rate has not improved, ventilation should be continued at a rate of 30–40 breaths/minute. The administration of naloxone should also be considered if narcotics were given in the last four hours before delivery. It is also worth checking again that the airway is clear.

Endotracheal intubation should be carried out if initial bag-and-mask ventilation has failed or if meconium aspiration is thought to have occurred in a baby that is not responding. A preterm baby may be difficult to resuscitate because an inadequate quantity of surfactant lining makes the lungs 'stiff'. By this time medical assistance should have arrived. Intubation is not difficult but needs to be undertaken by someone proficient in its use,[32] as intubation by an unskilled operator may be more dangerous than continuing effective mask ventilation.[26]

Neonatal asphyxia causes an imbalance in tissue oxygenation, causing acidosis. Ventilating the baby with adequate oxygen may enable it to establish respiration. If the heart is not adequately perfusing the tissues, chest compression will increase the heart rate so that oxygen permeates the cells throughout the body and stabilises metabolism. Chest compressions should not be commenced before ventilation.[32]

Cardiac compression

Throughout the ventilation procedure observation of the heart rate should continue. Auscultation of the heart rate should ideally be done with a stethoscope over the apex, but can also be easily felt with two fingers. Although pulsations can be felt at the base of the cord, these may not be reliable.

After the lungs have been aerated, if the heart rate is less than 60 beats per minute, chest compressions should commence. *See* Figure 2.12 for the recommended hand positions. The most effective method is gripping the chest with both hands, with the two thumbs opposed over the lower third of the sternum, just below an imaginary line joining the nipples, with the fingers over the spine at the baby's back. However, in some situations, usually when only one rescuer is present or due to lack of space, the two-finger method can be used (two fingers over the middle third of the sternum 1 cm below the nipple line). The compressions should aim to reduce the area from the chest to the spine by about one-third, and are done at a rate of about 140 compressions/minute. The ratio of three compressions to one breath should be maintained, ensuring that the chest rises with each breath.

Following the commencement of chest compression and ventilation, assessment of vital signs should be made regularly. If the heart rate continues to be below 60 beats per minute, the administration of drugs to stimulate the baby would be the next step. The insertion of a direct line via

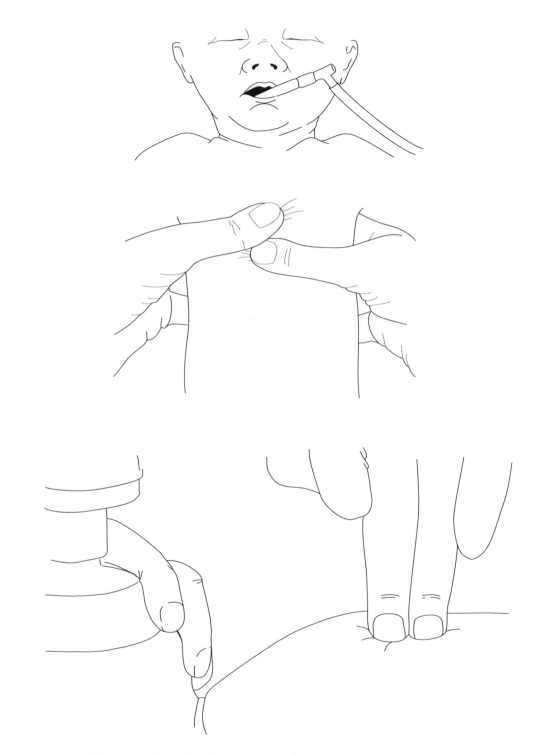

FIGURE 2.12 Finger positions for chest compression

BOX 2.10 Resuscitation equipment available in hospital

- A resuscitaire with a flat bed, an overhead heater, light, stethoscope and clock/timer. An apparatus fixed to the wall and available in the room may be preferable to a resuscitaire as it is less cumbersome and may be less frightening for the family.
- A supply of dry/warm towels
- Fluid chart
- Drug chart
- Infant's notes.

To maintain the airway
- Suction, not exceeding minus 100 mmHg
- Suction catheters in sizes 6, 8 and 10 FG
- Oropharyngeal airways in sizes 0 and 00
- Nasogastric tubes.

For ventilation
- Self-inflating bag and mask (Laerdal bag)
- Face masks in sizes 0/0 and 0/1
- T tubing
- Oxygen supply, tubing and related flow valves

- Intubation equipment:
  - laryngoscopes and duplicate blades in sizes 1 and 0, spare bulbs and batteries
  - tracheal tubes in sizes 2.5, 3.0, 3.5 and 4.0, with adapters
  - introducers
  - tape.

Drugs and intravenous fluids
- Intravenous access materials
- Adrenaline 1:10 000 solution
- Naloxone
- Vitamin K (Konakion®), 1 mg in 0.5 ml
- Dextrose 10%
- Sodium bicarbonate 4.2%. This is not generally used where basic life support is required following birth. It may be used once blood gases are available to balance an obviously unbalanced blood picture[32]
- Albumin 4.5%
- Sodium chloride 0.9%
- Water for injection
- Syringes, needles, three-way taps, infusion sets.

the umbilical vein or administration via an endotracheal tube are the best routes.

The equipment usually available in a hospital for neonatal resuscitation is listed in Box 2.10.

Planned home birth

In the planned home situation it is less usual to encounter problems in the newborn baby following a normal birth. Drugs are always minimally used and labour is usually normal and straightforward. It is a good principle to bear in mind that two midwives should attend a home birth, so one midwife can be responsible for the care of the baby, and the other for the mother. Since the need for resuscitation cannot always be anticipated, it would be good practice for resuscitation equipment to be assembled and laid out before the birth, to be easily accessible in case it is needed.

If necessary the midwife would immediately dry the baby, which would give stimulation, wrapping well in warm towels and administer oxygen, observing the heart rate and respiratory effort. A clear airway is essential, but it is important, as previously mentioned, that any suction is gentle. If immediate recovery does not take place, a call for emergency backup is vital. While this is coming, respiration should be assisted with a mask and bag, in the same way as described previously. Likewise, if the heart is beating at less than 60 beats per minute, chest compressions should be commenced at a 3:1 ratio.

Resuscitation at home is fraught with problems, including the lack of equipment (*see* Box 2.11 for essentials), isolation from advanced medical care and the eventual inevitable transfer to the hospital. However, a good outcome can nevertheless be achieved.[29,32]

BOX 2.11 Resuscitation equipment available at home births
- Portable suction (ideally battery and mains operated) with appropriate suction catheters
- Portable oxygen
- Bag and mask
- Good light and some form of heating
- Torch (ideally a 'headband' variety)
- Watch or clock with a second hand
- Stethoscope
- Warm towels
- Notes
- Printed emergency instruction cards to enable a helper to summon help effectively and efficiently.

Unexpected birth

In the event of birth taking place unexpectedly and where no resuscitation equipment is available, ventilation can be carried out by the midwife covering the baby's nose and mouth with her mouth and exhaling so that the newborn's chest moves. Cardiac compression will also be necessary if the baby's heart rate is less than 60 beats per minute, and this can be assessed by placing two fingers over the apex.

Record keeping

During the emergency, whether in hospital or not and despite the situation being tense and worrying, all events must be recorded accurately. In a hospital setting, where there is more likely to be additional help available, one midwife could take on the role of 'scribe'. At home, the second midwife jotting down times and actions when she is able to may act as a prompt when writing notes 'in retrospect'.

Outcomes and support

In the tension of the resuscitation situation the parents must not be forgotten. When there is silence after the delivery and the mother asks, 'Is my baby all right?' it can be difficult for the midwife to know how to answer. Good communication is the key to most situations in life and most especially in this one. Often in a hospital delivery room neither the parents nor the midwife can see what is happening at the resuscitaire or, in some cases, resuscitation is taking place outside the room. However, the midwife can give the mother some idea as to what the team is doing to help the baby. The father may wish to stay with his partner or observe the resuscitation and this can only be decided with the parents at the time. Discussion after the event will also be useful for both staff and parents.

If the baby is admitted to a neonatal intensive care unit or even transferred to another hospital, the midwife should ensure that photographs are taken as soon as possible and given to the parents. They should also see the baby as soon as possible to help the attachment process. There may be situations, particularly in preterm birth, where resuscitation has to be discontinued. Parents should be prepared by the neonatal staff as to the possible outcomes,[32,36,37] and of course ongoing support by the midwife will be vital.

Following a tragic outcome, or perhaps even an unexpected resuscitation, there should be a support network available for the staff involved, and all midwives should ensure they are involved in caring for their colleagues in times of need.

References

1 Soar J, Deakin C, Nolan J, *et al.* (2005) European Resuscitation Council Guidelines for Resuscitation 05 section 7: cardiac arrest in special circumstances. *Resuscitation.* 67(Suppl. 1): S135–70.

2 Bothamley J, Boyle M. (2009) *Medical Conditions Affecting Pregnancy and Childbirth.* Oxford: Radcliffe.

3 Lewis G, editor. (2007) *The Confidential Enquiry into Maternal and Child Health (CEMACH). Saving Mothers' Lives: reviewing maternal deaths to make motherhood safer – 2003–2005. The Seventh Report on Confidential Enquiries into Maternal Deaths in the United Kingdom.* London: CEMACH.

4 Hayashi RH. (2000) Obstetric collapse. In: Kean L, Baker PN, Edelstone DI, editors. *Best Practice in Labour Ward Management.* 1st ed. London: WB Saunders.

5 Resuscitation Council (UK). (2005) Resuscitation Guidelines: adult advanced life support. Available at: www.resus.org.uk

6 Madams M. (2008) Maternal resuscitation: how to resuscitate mothers who die. *Br J Midwif.* 16(6): 372–8.

7 Plaat F. (2008) Anaesthetic issues related to postpartum haemorrhage (excluding antishock garments). *Best Pract Res Clin Obstet Gynaecol.* 22(6): 1043–56.

8 Rankin J. (2005) The renal tract. In: Stables D, Rankin J. *Physiology in Childbearing.* 2nd ed. London: Elsevier.

9 McCunn M, Dutton R. (2000) End points of resuscitation: how much is enough? *Curr Opin Anaesthesiol.* 13(2): 147–53.

10 Blackburn S. (2007) *Maternal, Fetal and Neonatal Physiology: a clinical perspective.* 3rd ed. London: Elsevier.

11 Goodwin A, Pearce A. (1992) The human wedge. *Anaesthesia,* 47: 433–4.

12 Bobrowski R. (2006) Trauma. In: James D, Steer P, Weiner C, Gonik B, editors. *High Risk pregnancy: management options.* 3rd ed. Philadelphia: Elsevier, Saunders.

13 Robson S. (2008) Medical care and medical disorders. In: Robson SE, Waugh J, *Medical Disorders in Pregnancy.* Oxford: Blackwell.

14 Resuscitation Council (UK). (2005) Resuscitation Guidelines: Adult Basic Life Support. Available at: www.resus.org.uk

15 Safar P. (1999) Ventilation and cardiopulmonary resuscitation. *Curr Opin Anaesthesiol.* 12(2): 165–71.

16 Billington M, Stevenson M. (2007) Anaesthesia and resuscitation of the critically ill woman. In: Billington M, Stevenson M, editors. *Critical Care in Childbirth for Midwives.* Oxford: Blackwell.

17 Peerless J. (2001) Fluid management of the trauma patient. *Curr Opin Anaesthesiol.* 14(2): 221–5.

18 Whitten M, Irvine L. (2000) Post-mortem and peri-mortem caesarean section: what are the indications? *J R Soc Med.* 93: 6–9.

19 Morris S, Stacey M. (2003) ABC of resuscitation: resuscitation in pregnancy. *BMJ.* 7426: 1277–9.

20 Boyd R. (2000) Witnessed resuscitation by relatives. *Resuscitation.* 43(3): 171–6.

21 Williams K. (1996) Witnessing resuscitation can help relatives. *Nurs Stand.* 11(3): 12.

22 Rattrie E. (2000) Witnessed resuscitation: good practice or not? *Nurs Stand.* 14(24): 32–5.

23 Adams S. (1994) Should relatives be allowed to watch resuscitation: a sister's experience. *BMJ.* 308(6945): 1687.

24 Kidby J. (2003) Family-witnessed cardiopulmonary resuscitation. *Nurs Stand.* 17(51): 33–6.

25 Maternal and Child Health Research Consortium. (2000) *Confidential Enquiry into Stillbirths and Deaths in Infancy (Seventh Annual Report)*. London: Maternal and Child Health Research Consortium.

26 Marlow N, Baker P. (2006) Resuscitation and immediate care of the newborn. In: James D, Steer P, Weiner C, Gonik B, editors. *High Risk Pregnancy: management options*. 3rd ed. Philadelphia: Elsevier, Saunders.

27 Johnson MH, Everitt BJ. (2001) *Essential Reproduction*. 5th ed. Oxford: Blackwell Scientific.

28 Novak B. (2005) Adaptation to extrauterine life: respiration and cardiovascular function. In: Stables D, Rankin J. *Physiology in Childbearing*. 2nd ed. London: Elsevier.

29 Drew D, Jevon P, Raby M. (2000) *Resuscitation of the Newborn: a practical approach*. Oxford: Butterworth Heinemann.

30 Ehrenstein V, Pedersen L, Grijota M, *et al.* (2009) Association of Apgar score at five minutes with long-term neurologic disability and cognitive function in a prevalence study of Danish conscripts. *BMC Pregnancy and Childbirth*. 9(14).

Available at: www.biomedcentral.com/content/pdf/1471-2393-9-14.pdf

31 Casey B, McIntire D, Leveno K. (2001) The continuing value of the Apgar score for the assessment of newborn infants. *N Engl J Med*. 344(7): 467–71.

32 International Liaison Committee on Resuscitation. (2000) Neonatal resuscitation. *Resuscitation*. 46: 401–16.

33 Vain N, Szyld E, Prudent L, *et al.* (2004) Oropharyngeal and nasopharyngeal suctioning of meconium-stained neonates before delivery of their shoulders: multicentre, randomized controlled trial. *Lancet*. 364: 597–602.

34 Halliday HL. (2001) Endotracheal intubation at birth for preventing morbidity and mortality in vigorous, meconium-stained infants born at term. *Cochrane Database Syst Rev*. 1: CD000500.

35 Resuscitation Council (UK). (2005) *Resuscitation Guidelines: newborn life support*. Available at: www.resus.org.uk.

36 Soll R. (1999) Consensus and controversy over resuscitation of the newborn infant. *Lancet*. 354(9172): 4–5.

37 McHaffie H. (1998) Withdrawing treatment from neonates: a review of the issues. *Br J Midwif*. 6(6): 384–8.

CHAPTER 3

Thromboembolism in pregnancy

Judy Bothamley

Introduction

Pulmonary thromboembolism is responsible for up to 12 maternal deaths a year and remains the leading direct cause of maternal mortality in the UK and the second most common cause of maternal death overall.[1] Pulmonary embolism (PE) occurs when a clot from a deep vein, commonly in the leg, detaches itself and travels to the lungs where it lodges in a pulmonary blood vessel. Collapse and death will occur if the clot is large enough to compromise the pulmonary circulation. Pregnancy is a hypercoagulable state, making pregnant women more prone to developing the deep vein thrombosis (DVT) that underlies this disorder. Prevention, detection and treatment of a DVT are crucial in limiting deaths from PE in pregnancy and the postpartum period. The management of a DVT, therefore, although not constituting an emergency of itself, will be discussed fully in this chapter alongside the immediate diagnosis and treatment of a woman presenting with a PE. Midwives have an important role in risk assessment for venous thromboembolism (VTE) so that those women at risk can be identified and appropriate preventative measures taken.

Epidemiology

VTE (which includes DVT and PE) is up to 10 times more common in pregnant women compared to non-pregnant women of a similar age.[2–4] Difficulty in making a definitive diagnosis and lack of national reporting makes estimation of the incidence of VTE difficult. In a recent, large (n=613 232) register-based study from Norway the overall incidence of VTE was found to be 1 per 1000 pregnancies.[5] VTE can occur at any time during the childbearing period and similar numbers present in the antenatal period as the postnatal period.[2,5] However, when considering that the antenatal period extends over a much longer time period (40 weeks) compared to the postnatal period (six weeks) the daily risk of VTE in the postpartum period is much higher.[6] It can also be noted that approximately 40% of VTE in pregnancy occur in the first trimester, indicating that the procoagulant changes that occur in pregnancy start early.[7]

Of VTE events that occur in association with childbearing about 80% are DVT and 20% are PE.[8] Timely diagnosis of DVT is essential in preventing deaths from PE as a PE will develop in about a quarter of women with undiagnosed and untreated DVT.[9] Two-thirds of deaths from pulmonary embolism may occur within 30 minutes of the embolic event. In the recent report, *The Confidential Enquiry into Maternal and Child Health (CEMACH), Saving Mother's Lives*, 33 women died of PE with 10 of these deaths occurring during the first trimester. Fifteen women died postnatally, eight following vaginal delivery and seven after caesarean section.[1] In order to gather data about non-fatal PE, a national case-controlled study of antenatal pulmonary embolism was undertaken through the United Kingdom Obstetric Surveillance System (UKOSS). This study determined the antenatal incidence of PE to be 13.1 per 100 000.[10] Figures for non-fatal postnatal PE in the UK are currently not available but extrapolation from the Norwegian study[5] would suggest a rate of approximately 22 per 100 000.

Pathophysiology

Clot formation normally occurs in response to injury in a vessel wall and is an important mechanism to prevent blood loss. It is a complex process involving a cascade of reactions whereby fibrinogen, a soluble protein in the blood, is converted to produce fibrin threads, by the action of thrombin. Blood cells attach to the fibrin threads and clump together to form a clot. A DVT will develop when small deposits of fibrin collect in the leg veins (often thigh or calf veins) as a result of slow blood flow. They may occur around the cusp of a venous valve, which can cause irreversible valve damage, resulting in chronic valve insufficiency and a condition known as post-thrombotic syndrome. PE occurs when the clot extends and breaks off, travelling through the venous system to the lungs where it lodges in a pulmonary blood vessel, which obstructs blood flow to the lungs. Symptoms of PE will vary depending on how much the pulmonary circulation and consequently oxygen exchange is affected (*see* section on PE later in this chapter).

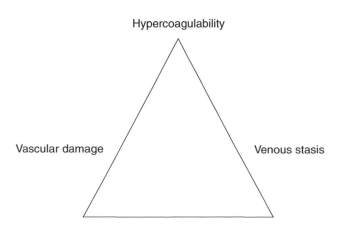

FIGURE 3.1 Triad of factors associated with venous thrombosis

Rudolf Virchow (1821–1902) first described the triad of factors that are associated with venous thrombosis, all of which are present during pregnancy and the puerperium (*see* Figure 3.1)[4,11]

Hypercoagulability

Normal pregnancy is associated with alterations in the proteins of the coagulation and fibrinolytic systems, resulting in a relative state of hypercoagulability.[3] These changes are an adaptive and preparatory mechanism for the control of bleeding in the third stage of labour and help maintain the placenta–uterine interface.[11] Procoagulant factors, such as von Willebrand factor, factor VIII, factor V and fibrinogen enhance thrombin production in pregnancy.[4] In addition, an acquired resistance to the anticoagulant protein C and a reduction in protein S further contribute to the increased coagulability. Impaired fibrinolysis, resulting in slower breakdown of clots, also occurs.[12]

Venous stasis

Venous return from the lower limbs is reduced when the pregnant uterus compresses the inferior vena cava. In addition, reduction in the muscle tone of veins during pregnancy, caused by progesterone, leads to vasodilation and reduced velocity of blood flow.[2,3,12] There can be up to a 50% reduction in blood flow (venous return) with peak effect occurring around 36 weeks' gestation and taking about six weeks postnatal to return to pre-pregnancy levels.[4,13] Blood remains in contact with the vessel wall for a longer time and this may be an important factor in the development of a DVT. Incompetent venous valves are a common source of morbidity in women of reproductive age and may also contribute to venous stasis.

Blood flow within the veins depends on the action of voluntary muscles and periods of inactivity further slow blood flow. The anatomy of the venous drainage from the lower limb, where the left iliac vein is crossed by the right iliac artery, means that DVTs are more common (more than 80%) in the left leg.[2,4]

Vascular damage

The venous epithelium is normally an intact, smooth, single layer of cells containing various substances to prevent platelet adhesion and clot formation. Trauma damaging the vessel wall will set off a series of chemical reactions that will allow platelet aggregation at the site of injury and fibrin formation which results in the development of a clot. Endothelial damage to pelvic vessels can occur during vaginal or operative delivery.[12]

Influential reports aimed at reducing deaths from PE in the UK

The triennial review of maternal deaths in the UK (Confidential Enquiries into Maternal Deaths [CEMD]) latterly produced by CEMACH (now known as Centre for Maternal and Child Enquiries, CMACE), has been influential in identifying factors that can contribute to limiting deaths from PE. Concern was highlighted over the number of deaths occurring following caesarean section and in response to this, in 1995, the Royal College of Obstetrics and Gynaecologists (RCOG) published recommendations for risk assessment and thromboprophylaxis following caesarean section,[13] which were widely adopted. The 2001 report of CEMD *Why Mothers Die 1997–1999*[14] noted a sharp fall in deaths following caesarean section; however, deaths following vaginal delivery had remained static. In response to this the RCOG produced guidelines that recommended risk assessment following vaginal delivery.[15] The need for risk assessment in the antenatal and even pre-conception period has featured in more recent CEMACH reports,[1,16] with a particular increased concern about obesity and greater awareness of thrombophilia. A number of studies examining risk factors for VTE over the last 10 years have been published so that effective risk assessment tools can be developed.[5,10,17] Guidance for reducing the risk of thromboembolism during pregnancy, birth and the puerperium with an emphasis on risk assessment has recently been published by the RCOG.[18] International guidelines regarding VTE in pregnancy have also been developed.[19]

Risk assessment

A consideration of risk factors in the context of individualised care is important in the prevention of thromboembolism. Most women who died from PE had identifiable risk factors and use of a risk assessment tool aims to improve identification, appropriate referral and improved management of women at risk of VTE. An assessment for risk factors for VTE should be made at booking, repeated if admitted to hospital and after/during delivery.[19] Ideally, those women with a high risk of VTE should access pre-conception advice as 'booking' often does not occur until the end of the first trimester, after the stage when thromboprophylaxis should have begun. General practitioners, physicians, other health professionals and the general public need to recognise the need for pre-conception planning for the woman at high risk of VTE.

BOX 3.1 Risk factors for VTE in pregnancy and the postpartum period[5,10,17,19–21]

General conditions
- Personal or family history of DVT, PE or thrombophilia
- Anticardiolipin antibodies (antiphospholipid syndrome or as part of systemic lupus erythematosus)
- Inherited thrombophilias, e.g. Factor V Leiden
- Age over 35
- Obesity (BMI >30)
- Prolonged immobilisation, e.g. paraplegia
- Major current illness, e.g. heart, lung, kidney or bowel disease, malignancy
- Sickle-cell disease
- Long-distance air travel
- Major varicose veins
- Smoking
- Combined oral contraceptive pill.

Pregnancy-related factors
- Caesarean section
- Parity ≥three[19]/parity >one[10]
- Multiple pregnancies
- Assisted reproduction
- Severe infection
- Pre-eclampsia
- Immobility (including bedrest, symphysis pubis dysfunction)
- Surgical procedures in pregnancy
- Prolonged labour, instrumental delivery
- Ovarian hyperstimulation syndrome
- Dehydration, hyperemesis
- Excessive blood loss.

The midwife at the booking interview already gathers the required information (such as smoking, BMI, previous medical or family history of VTE), required for

Antenatal assessment and management (to be assessed at booking and repeated if admitted)

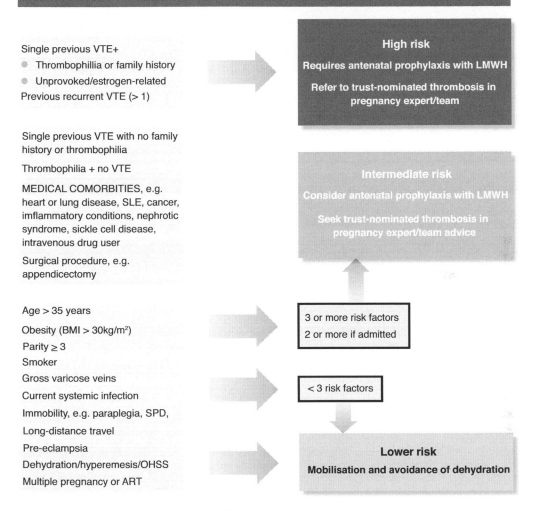

Antenatal and postnatal prophylactic dose of LMWH

Weight <50 kg - 20 mg enoxaparin/2500 units dalteparin/3500 units tinzaparin daily

Weight 50-90 kg - 40 mg enoxaparin/5000 units dalteparin/4500 units tinzaparin daily

Weight 91-130 kg - 60 mg enoxaparin/7500 units dalteparin/7000 units tinzaparin daily

Weight 131-170 kg - 80 mg enoxaparin/10000 units dalteparin/9000 units tinzaparin daily

Weight >170 kg - 0.6 mg/kg/day enoxaparin: 75 units/kg/day dalteparin/75 units/kg/day tinzaparin

Key

ART - assisted reproductive therapy, BMI - body mass index (based on booking weight), gross varicose veins - symptomatic, above the knee or associated with phlebitis/oedema/skin changes, immobility - ≥ 3 days, LMWH - low-molecular-weight heparin, OHSS - ovarian hyperstimulation syndrome, PPH - postpartum haemorrhage, SLE - systemic lupus erythematosus, SPD - symphysis pubis dysfunction with reduced mobility, thrombophilia - inherited or acquired, long-distance travel - > 4 hours, VTE - venous thromboembolism

FIGURE 3.2 Antenatal assessment and management (reproduced with the permission of the RCOG)

Postnatal assessment and management (to be assessed on delivery suite)

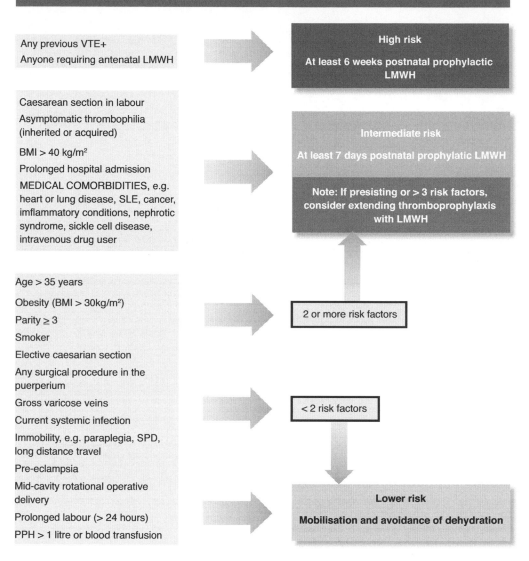

Key

ART – assisted reproductive therapy, BMI – body mass index (based on booking weight), gross varicose veins – symptomatic, above the knee or associated with phlebitis/oedema/skin changes, immobility – ≥ 3 days, LMWH - low-molecular-weight heparin, OHSS – ovarian hyperstimulation syndrome, PPH – postpartum haemorrhage, SLE – systemic lupus erythematosus, SPD – symphysis pubis dysfunction with reduced mobility, thrombophilia – inherited or acquired, long-distance travel – > 4 hours, VTE – venous thrombo embolism

FIGURE 3.3 Postnatal assessment and management (reproduced with the permission of the RCOG)

risk assessment of VTE[17] so completion of a risk assessment tool should not be onerous. Box 3.1 lists the risk factors commonly identified to be associated with VTE. The risk assessment tool devised by the RCOG 2009[19] is reproduced with permission as Figures 3.2 and 3.3.

Those women considered high risk should receive, or be considered for, antenatal thromboprophylaxis with *low molecular weight heparin* (LMWH) (*see* section on anticoagulation treatment and prevention of DVT and PE later in this chapter). Where identified this should commence as early in pregnancy as practically possible (in view of increased first trimester risk). The midwife needs to identify these women and make timely and efficient referral to the appropriate medical practitioner to ensure this occurs. Some high-risk women may not require prophylaxis in the antenatal period but will require it in the postnatal period as the postnatal period is a time of enhanced daily risk.

Women should be risk assessed again following delivery to determine the need for postnatal prophylaxis with LMWH and for how long they should receive it (*see* Figure 3.3). It appears the prothrombotic changes of pregnancy do not resolve until some weeks after delivery. Those at high risk of VTE in the postnatal period are recommended thromboprophylaxis for six weeks. Some women may change to the oral anticoagulant warfarin about a week after delivery if they were taking maintenance doses of warfarin before pregnancy. There is some uncertainty with regard to optimal duration of LMWH thromboprophylaxis for those women at intermediate risk. Recent guidance recommends LMWH thromboprophylaxis for seven days postpartum in this group of women.[19] Midwives should ensure all women, regardless of risk, mobilise and avoid dehydration during and following delivery (*see* section on 'Medical and midwifery measures to prevent VTE').

BOX 3.2 Women that will be considered for antenatal prophylaxis with LMWH

- Those with previous VTE – this may have been while on oestrogen-containing contraception, in a previous pregnancy, associated with prior surgery or as an unprovoked event.
- Those with three or more risk factors (*see* Box 3.1) or two or more if admitted to hospital.
- Those with diagnosis of inherited or acquired thrombophilia and/or family history of VTE in first-degree relative.

Risk factors
Inherited or acquired thrombophilia

An alteration in the balance between the coagulation and fibrinolytic systems caused by inherited or acquired disorders predisposes a woman to clot formation. Genetic or acquired disorders are linked to approximately half of pregnancy-related VTE,[22] although many women with thrombophilia don't develop thrombosis complications, indicating that the development of VTE is multicausal. Examples of thrombophilia disorders are listed in Box 3.3.

Having multiple thrombophilia, homozygous defects and particular high-risk thrombophilia (such as APS) will increase overall risk for VTE in pregnancy.[20,23] Universal screening for thrombophilia in pregnancy is not recommended as tests are technically difficult due to procoagulant changes in pregnancy[19] and thought not to be cost effective.[26] Thrombophilia is associated with other pregnancy risks in addition to VTE including recurrent and late fetal loss, pre-eclampsia, placental abruption and intrauterine growth restriction.[24,27]

Referral for specialist medical advice (ideally before pregnancy) is recommended for women with clinical features that suggest the possibility of thrombophilia (*see* Box 3.4).

Previous history of VTE

Not surprisingly, a previous history of VTE increases the risk for thromboembolism in pregnancy and the postnatal period, in the region of 10%–14%.[3] Women who have had a VTE would ideally have been screened for congenital thrombophilia prior to pregnancy. The midwife should refer these women to an obstetrician/ physician/haematologist as appropriate so that a plan of management can be determined.

Obesity

The CEMACH report *Saving Mother's Lives*[1] noted that 50% of the women who died, for which a BMI was recorded, were obese. With significant and rising prevalence of obesity in the childbearing population this is an important risk factor for VTE in pregnancy and this risk appears to increase with rising BMI.[28]

Inadequate anticoagulation caused by maternal weight not being taken into account when heparin was prescribed has been implicated, and guidance for weight-related thromboprophylactic and treatment dose of LMWH are included in guidance from RCOG.[19] Immobility associated with obesity (with consequent venous stasis), increased complications of childbirth generally[29] and use of the combined oral contraceptive pill[30] postnatally are all cofactors contributing to the risk of VTE in obese women.

Pre-eclampsia

Pre-eclampsia is associated with vascular injury, which in turn is related to a disturbance in coagulation, thereby suggesting a link with thromboembolism. Confounding factors, such as caesarean section and bedrest, may contribute to the risk of thromboembolism in women with pre-eclampsia. Van Walraven *et al.*[31] suggest that thrombophilia may cause clots to form in placental blood vessels, predisposing women to development of pre-eclampsia and explaining the link between pre-eclampsia and VTE.

Immobility

Movement of calf muscles and deep respiratory effort promote venous return and prevent stasis. Most pregnant women are healthy and active, but there are occasions when they become less mobile and are susceptible to thromboembolism. Changes in patterns of antenatal and postnatal care have contributed to the avoidance of bedrest for pregnant women and probably account for the overall reduction in thromboembolism over the years. However, bedrest does occur after caesarean section and at a time of severe pre-eclampsia. Bedrest, as a treatment for premature labour and premature rupture of membranes, was associated with an increase in thromboembolism.[32] Admission to hospital with hyperemesis combines the risk effects of immobilisation and dehydration.

The CEMACH report *Saving Mother's Lives*[1] reported the deaths of two pregnant women following air travel. Increased venous stasis caused by pressure on the back of the calves from prolonged sitting, low atmospheric pressure and dehydration may all contribute to increased risk of VTE. Long-haul travel of any kind is included in the RCOG risk assessment tool (*see* Figure 3.2). Guidance on air travel in pregnancy has been published by the RCOG.[33]

The CEMD report published in 1998[34] included a paraplegic woman who died of PE in the postnatal period. Overcoming the problems of immobility for these women

represents a particular challenge. More recently symphysis pubis dysfunction has been identified as another possible cause for sustained immobility in pregnancy.[35]

Medical and midwifery measures to prevent VTE

There are a number of medical and midwifery measures that can be introduced to help prevent VTE, with the midwife playing an important role in educating women, administering medication, fitting thromboembolic deterrent (TED) stockings and detecting signs and symptoms of DVT and PE. Box 3.5 lists common prophylactic measures to prevent DVT.

Thromboembolic deterrent stockings (TEDS)

TEDS, also known as graduated compression stockings, aim to promote venous return, decrease leg swelling and prevent primary and recurrent DVT. External compression increases the velocity of blood flow within the veins, reducing venous stasis.[36] While clinical data on the effect of stockings in preventing DVT in pregnancy is lacking, evidence of an improvement in venous haemodynamics of the legs during pregnancy and the postpartum period has been shown.[37] It seems reasonable that the benefits shown in non-pregnant individuals would also apply in pregnancy. They may be used in conjunction with LMWH, for women where LMWH is contraindicated and for women travelling by air. Their use is also advocated to decrease the risk and severity of post-thrombotic syndrome, a condition caused by damage to venous valves. Post-thrombotic syndrome varies from mild oedema to incapacitating swelling with pain and ulceration, and

BOX 3.5 Prophylactic measures that may be used to prevent thromboembolism

For those at higher risk (see Figures 3.2 and 3.3)

- Thromboprophylaxis with prescribed LMWH.

Generally as indicated, and for those with additional risk factors

- Avoiding long period of immobilisation
- Wearing correctly fitting thromboembolic deterrent (TED) stockings
- Deep-breathing exercises to encourage venous return
- Effective postpartum pain relief to enable mobility

- Intermittent pneumatic compression system during operative procedures.[38]

General measures for all pregnant women

- Do leg exercises to encourage venous return.
- Drink plenty of water and avoid dehydration.
- Avoid sitting with legs crossed.
- Avoid prolonged immobilisation.
- Take regular breaks on long journeys.
- Seek specific advice about air travel in pregnancy.

early application of TED stockings in patients and pregnant women with acute DVT may prevent this complication.

There is lack of data with regards to pregnancy about which length stocking (knee or thigh) offers greater benefit. Reviews on the non-pregnant population suggest knee-length stockings were effective, cheaper, more likely to fit correctly and better tolerated by the people wearing them.[39,40]

Accurate fitting of stockings may be more difficult in pregnancy due to changing levels of oedema. However, the RCOG (2009)[19] recommends the use of properly applied thigh-length TED with knee-length being considered if full length are ill fitting or when compliance is poor. Many women may not wear them because they find them uncomfortable and/or don't understand the need for them.[41] Box 3.6 outlines guidance for correct use of TED stockings.

BOX 3.6 Guidance for correct use of TED stockings[41,42]

- Use manufacturer's instructions for measuring, selecting correct size and fitting stockings.
- Apply carefully, ensuring toe hole lies under toes, the heel patch is in correct position and the thigh gusset is over the inner thigh.
- Stockings should be smooth when fitted. Ensure they don't roll down, which gives a tourniquet effect.
- Remove daily for no more than 30 minutes.
- Check fitting daily to detect changes in leg circumference.
- Advise women how they work and why they can help reduce DVT along with advice about how to wear them.

Prophylaxis for pregnant women travelling by air

Precautionary measures to avoid DVT are recommended for pregnant women travelling by air. These include leg and ankle exercises, walking around the cabin when possible, avoiding dehydration by drinking plenty of non-alcoholic drinks and by minimising alcohol and caffeine intake and the wearing of correctly fitting TED stockings.[1,2] Women at high risk of DVT should discuss specific prophylaxis measures with an obstetrician/ physician.[33]

Deep vein thrombosis
Diagnosis of DVT

The diagnosis of DVT in pregnancy is difficult. Signs and symptoms (*see* Box 3.7) will raise suspicion of a DVT, but only a small percentage will have the diagnosis confirmed.[43]

BOX 3.7 Symptoms and signs of DVT[2,11,44]

- Pain in calf, thigh, groin, buttocks (especially unilateral pain)
- Swelling (at least 2 cm difference between the two legs)
- Redness or discoloration of the affected leg
- Change in limb colour or temperature
- Homan's sign (pain on dorsiflexion of the foot) (unreliable)
- Low-grade pyrexia (37.5°C)
- Tachycardia (pulse 100/min)
- Lower abdominal pain
- Limb symptoms on left side (80%)
- Chest pain and shortness of breath (symptoms of PE).

The general discomfort and swelling of a woman's legs in pregnancy can confuse the diagnosis, and assessment should be made in context of additional risk factors. DVTs in pregnancy may not be in the calf vein but higher up in the ileofemoral region. The higher the location of the clot, the more likely it is to cause a PE and the more difficult it is to be seen on ultrasound. Confusingly, lower abdominal pain associated with clots in higher level veins can be the presenting feature of DVT in pregnancy.[11] Ovarian vein thrombosis, which is more likely on the right side, presents with flank, back or groin pain. Cerebral venous thrombosis may present as severe headaches.[2] The latter are very rare. Referral to a senior obstetrician and careful evaluation of additional risk factors form an essential part of the clinical assessment of a woman presenting with symptoms of DVT.

Diagnostic tests for DVT

Accurate diagnosis is essential, not only to prevent PE but also to protect women from unnecessary treatment with anticoagulants. *Compression ultrasound* is the primary diagnostic test for detecting DVT in pregnancy. When thrombus is present, a relatively echogenic soft tissue mass, which prevents the vein collapsing after compression of the leg, is seen. The calf veins and veins above the inguinal ligament may not be clearly seen with this technique. For calf veins ultrasound is repeated after seven days to see if the clot has extended. When results are equivocal, or a higher level thrombosis is suspected, venography (injection of contrast medium), may be used.[2,43] *Fibrin degradation products (D-dimers)* are formed as a thrombus develops and can be measured in the blood to raise suspicion of a DVT. D-dimer assays are commonly used in conjunction with ultrasound in non-pregnant patients. However, false positives are common, especially in late pregnancy, and are of no clinical value in the postpartum period.[2] Low levels of D-dimer in pregnancy are likely, as in non-pregnant patients, to suggest that there is no thrombus, although a recent case report suggests unreliability even in this circumstance.[45]

Management of DVT

Treatment with LMWH is recommended where DVT or PE is suspected by clinical assessment until proven otherwise by diagnostic tests.[46] In addition to anticoagulation other interventions that will aid recovery are aimed at promoting good venous return, thereby preventing further clot formation. Leg elevation is recommended when sitting, but in pregnancy inguinal congestion may occur, so the leg should not be raised at too acute an angle and pressure behind the knee should be avoided. Once anticoagulants have been commenced and full-length TED stockings fitted (*see* section on thromboembolic deterrent stockings), mobility is encouraged.[12,46]

General measures to prevent DVT (*see* Box 3.5) should be emphasised. Midwives should provide women with information about DVT and how to prevent further clot formation as well as inform them about signs and symptoms of PE and when to seek further medical aid. The RCOG has produced a helpful leaflet *Venous Thrombosis in Pregnancy and After Birth. Information for You.*[47]

Pulmonary embolism

The clinical signs of PE (*see* Box 3.8) are related to the size of the clot that is obstructing the pulmonary circulation. Large or multiple emboli will prevent adequate oxygenation of the blood. A woman with a major PE will collapse with severe breathlessness, cyanosis, hypotension and chest pain. Sudden respiratory or cardiac arrest may occur.

Warning signs and symptoms indicative of smaller emboli include unexplained pyrexia, cough, chest pain and breathlessness, which may be incorrectly diagnosed as a chest infection. An infective cause for these symptoms should only be considered after a PE has been excluded. Breathlessness, rapid breathing and leg discomfort occur commonly as pregnancy progresses and consequently might be ignored.

BOX 3.8 Clinical manifestations of PE[2,44]

Most frequent signs and symptoms

- Sudden or unexpected difficulty in breathing
- Increased respiratory rate (tachypnoea)
- Feeling faint
- Tightness in chest or pleuritic chest pain
- Increased pulse (tachycardia)
- Cough
- Crackles on auscultation.

Associated signs and symptoms

- Coughing up blood (haemoptysis)
- Distended neck veins
- Cyanosis and collapse
- Anxiety
- Low grade fever.

Assessed in combination with signs and symptoms of DVT

Diagnostic tools for PE

Assessment of the woman's condition will be undertaken with a chest X-ray, an ECG and tests of oxygen levels (saturation and blood gases) and although this will not lead to a diagnosis, the findings may identify other aetiologies and underpin treatment. A *chest X-ray* will identify other causes for chest symptoms such as pneumonia as well as show changes that may be indicative of PE. The radiation dose from chest X-ray is negligible, particularly as compared to other more definitive tests for PE (see below). If the X-ray is normal, examination of the legs by ultrasound scan (USS) is suggested as a diagnosis of DVT will indirectly confirm diagnosis of PE. If both chest X-ray and USS are negative but clinical concern is high, a *ventilation/perfusion (V/Q) scan* or *computed tomography pulmonary angiogram* (CTPA) should be performed.[46]

A *V/Q scan* consists initially of assessment of the pulmonary blood flow following an intravenous injection of albumin labelled with radioactive technetium.[46] Areas with reduced or absent perfusion are diagnostic of PE. The ventilation component of the V/Q scan increases the sensitivity of identifying underperfused and under-ventilated areas by collecting information regarding the distribution of inhaled gas. This component may be omitted in pregnancy to reduce radiation exposure to the fetus.[46] PE typically produces poor perfusion in an area of normal ventilation.[2]

A *CTPA* can be used, in which the chest is assessed using CT following the injection of a dye into the bloodstream; however, there is a higher radiation dose to the breasts compared to a V/Q scan, which may increase lifetime risk of breast cancer.[4,46] Using breast shields will reduce exposure.[4] In addition, *in utero* radiation exposure may increase the risk of childhood cancer.[4,46] Overall, the risk of death from untreated PE clearly outweighs the risks of radiation exposure. Clinicians need to aim to reduce the number of tests performed while still attaining accurate diagnosis.[4] The implications of both these tests should be discussed fully with the woman and informed consent obtained.

Treatment of pulmonary embolism

Early diagnosis and treatment is vital when PE is suspected, as deaths caused by PE can occur very quickly following an embolic event. A woman presenting with massive pulmonary embolus may suffer cardiovascular collapse. Appropriate staff, including a senior anaesthetist and physician, should be urgently summoned to deal with this emergency or if the woman is at home, she should be immediately transferred to the closest accident and emergency department via ambulance. The surgical team and a radiologist may also be required.

Immediate treatment should include standard assessment, with the commencement of continuous vital-sign measurement as well as ECG, intravenous access and oxygen therapy. An urgent echocardiogram or CT pulmonary angiogram (CTPA) needs to be arranged. Cardiac arrest procedures, including endotracheal intubation and mechanical ventilation, may be required.[46] If the woman is making some respiratory effort it is advisable to put the head of the bed up by 30 degrees and/or assist her to lean forwards to help maximise lung expansion along with delivery of oxygen via face mask. If the cause of the collapse is thought likely to be PE, LMWH or intravenous unfractionated heparin should be started immediately[4] and given according to local guidelines (*see* section on anti-coagulation treatment and prevention of DVT and PE). The midwife should provide the necessary support to the anaesthetist, physician and/or obstetrician in instigating these therapies.

Other specific midwifery management includes the assessment and documentation of respiratory and cardiovascular vital signs. Assessment of oxygen saturation levels will be made initially with an oximeter and then via arterial blood gas monitoring. Intravenous access will have been established as soon as possible and bloods taken (full blood count [FBC], coagulation and renal and liver function tests). Accurate recording of fluid balance, including hourly urine output after catheterisation, is important in preventing further insult to the cardiovascular system through fluid overload: a central venous pressure (CVP) or arterial line may be necessary.

The woman, if conscious, will be extremely apprehensive and agitated. A calm, confident, sympathetic approach by the midwife may help to minimise this apprehension. Members of the woman's family will also require support, guidance and information at the time and following this event. Midwifery staff may also need to take responsibility for the care of the newborn. Box 3.9 summarises the main responsibilities for the midwife, a number of which can be instigated in the home setting while emergency transfer to hospital is arranged.

Further medical or surgical interventions may be necessary in life-threatening pulmonary embolism. *Thrombolytic therapy* ('clot-busting' drugs such as streptokinase) may be used, but this is not common in pregnancy except in a life-threatening situation, due to the risk of major haemorrhage and fetal loss.[4,48] In cases where recurring clots are developing, *inferior vena cava filters*, which work by intercepting emboli travelling to the pulmonary vasculature, have been used safely in pregnancy.[49] *Pulmonary embolectomy* is rarely used, but *pulmonary angiography*, with the use of a guideline wire via a cardiac catheter, may be successful in breaking up the clot, although there is a high radiation exposure.[46]

BOX 3.9 Midwife's responsibilities in pulmonary embolism emergency

- Summon the emergency response team or arrange emergency transfer by ambulance to hospital if at home.
- Administer CPR if necessary.
- Assist with endotracheal intubation as necessary.
- Give oxygen.
- If appropriate, sit the woman up to maximise the respiratory effort.
- Initiate IV access.
- Take blood for FBC, coagulation screen, urea, electrolytes and liver function tests.
- Assess and record cardiovascular and respiratory vital signs.
- Attach oximeter and record ECG.
- Give heparin and other drugs according to medical orders.
- Maintain accurate fluid balance.
- Monitor fetal well-being as appropriate.
- Support the woman and her family.
- Maintain accurate records.

Following any thromboembolic event, anticoagulation maintenance is used and continued for several weeks through pregnancy and the puerperium. This may involve regular monitoring. Anticoagulants commonly used are not contraindicated in breast feeding, but individual drugs should always be checked. Midwives may be involved in teaching women to give their daily injections, advise about side-effects such as bleeding from gums and bruising, and generally provide ongoing support following what may have been a very frightening experience.

Anticoagulation treatment and prevention of DVT and PE

Anticoagulation treatment aims to prevent extension of the clot, restore venous patency and limit the risk or recurrence of a PE. *Low molecular weight heparin* (LMWH) has largely replaced *unfractionated (standard) heparin* (UH) in the prevention and treatment of VTE in pregnancy. Unfractionated (standard) heparin can be administered via the intravenous (IV) or subcutaneous route. It is now mostly used only in acute treatment of major PE with cardiac and/or renal compromise. Midwives should familiarise themselves with local guidelines for intravenous heparin use in acute events.

Heparin (both LMWH and UH) doesn't break down a clot but prevents further clot formation by enhancing the action of antithrombin, which allows time for the normal process of fibrinolysis to break down the clot.[2] Heparin is a large molecule that does not cross the placenta, so the risk of teratogenesis or bleeding in the fetus is minimal. It is therefore considered safe for use during pregnancy and lactation.[50] Anticoagulation therapy can be influenced by renal and liver function. As conditions such as pre-eclampsia

may affect renal and liver function, blood should be tested for full blood count, coagulation screen, urea, electrolytes and liver function tests. Heparin-induced thrombocytopaenia is rare, but the platelet count should be rechecked at 5–14 days after the start of heparin therapy and monthly thereafter. The drug protamine can be used to reverse the effects of heparin.[4]

The last 20 years have seen the development of LMWH. There are several LMWHs, but the most commonly used in pregnancy are enoxaparin (Clexane®) and dalteparin (Fragmin®).[50] LMWH is administered by subcutaneous injection. It has several advantages over UH, including a longer half-life (therefore enabling once-daily injections) and less incidence of heparin-induced thrombocytopaenia and osteopaenia[50] and less need for laboratory monitoring. LMWH is commonly used for prophylaxis or in the chronic phase of treatment, but authorities now say that LMWH is also safe and effective for treatment of acute thromboembolism in pregnancy.[50,51] The therapeutic dose of LMWHs is maternal weight dependent.[19]

The risk of developing an epidural haematoma in women taking LMWH causes concern for anaesthetists.[2] In addition there may be a risk of bleeding, particularly in the third stage of labour, although evidence has been reassuring with regard to these risks.[50] Women taking LMWH maintenance therapy need to be advised not to give their scheduled injection once labour begins and will need to be assessed (including a coagulation screen) on admission to hospital. If delivery is planned, LMWH should be discontinued 24 hours before the planned delivery.[46] Clark[43] suggests epidural insertion should not be carried out within 12 hours of a prophylactic dose of LMWH and within 24 hours after a therapeutic dose. Midwives also need to be aware of the anaesthetist's instructions and local policies regarding the timing of removal of an epidural catheter in relation to LMWH injections. Midwives need to be proactive in ensuring good verbal and written communication between the woman, midwife, obstetrician and anaesthetist in this situation to enable best possible choices in pain relief to be available to this woman, balanced against the need to prevent VTE. General measures to promote venous return and prevent VTE such as mobilisation, leg exercises and preventing dehydration will be even more important to the woman who is at risk of VTE.

Warfarin is an oral anticoagulant and in contrast to heparin crosses the placenta, with particular risk of damage to the embryo if taken between six and 12 weeks' gestation. It is also associated with an increased risk of fetal loss even when first trimester exposure is avoided.[4] In addition, if taken around the time of delivery it can lead to bleeding in the neonate and it increases the risk of post-partum haemorrhage in the mother.[52] It may be used in the postpartum period as an alternative to LMWH. Regular assessment of the international normalised ratio (INR) is necessary, particularly in the first 10 days of treatment, which can prove inconvenient for the newly delivered mother. Warfarin does cross into the breast milk but has been shown not to impact the newborn's coagulation profile.[4] Women with prosthetic heart valves may be taking warfarin prior to pregnancy and a plan in consultation with a cardiologist is needed before pregnancy on how best to maintain effective anticoagulation balanced against risk to the fetus.

Midwifery responsibilities
Education, advice and support for women on anticoagulant treatment
Women generally show initial reluctance to give themselves heparin injections and the midwife should work through the requirements with the woman to develop her confidence. A clear incentive

TABLE 3.1 Laboratory tests for monitoring heparin[53]

Assay	Nature of the test	Comments
Activated partial thromboplastin time (APTT)	Measures time to clot formation after adding an activating agent	Can be difficult to measure and unpredictable in pregnancy
		Used to monitor effect of heparin on coagulation
Protamine titration (PT)	Determines the plasma level of heparin	
International normalised ratio (INR)	Thrombin is added to the plasma and time to clot recorded	Used to monitor blood clotting in people who take warfarin
Anti-factor Xa assay	Measures the rate of factor-Xa inhibition by optical density determination	Expensive; LMWH-specific; not widely available

to achieving self-management will be the possibility of discharge from hospital. Heparin, either unfractionated or LMWH, involves only small volumes, which are pre-loaded, and given with a fine-gauge needle. The site of subcutaneous injection should rotate between thighs and abdominal wall. Grasping some flesh, the injection is made at right angles to the skin surface. Bruising inevitably occurs at the site of injection. The woman should take care to take precautions in situations that may cause bleeding or injury; for example, a soft bristle toothbrush will protect from bleeding gums. Arrangements for safe disposal of needles should be made.

A phone call or visit from the midwife within days of discharge from hospital may be timely to offer support to the woman as she comes to terms with what will be prolonged treatment. A discussion regarding the management of any future pregnancies should be made at an appropriate time, probably after delivery, and in conjunction with the physician. The woman's risk of recurrent DVT and the use of the combined contraceptive pill should be discussed.

Similarly, those women being discharged from the hospital postnatally on prophylactic dose LMWH will need similar support and instruction. With implementation of the new guidelines published from the RCOG,[19] which advises LMWH prophylaxis for at least seven days following emergency caesarean section (CS) and also for those following elective CS who have additional risk factors (such as age over 35 and BMI greater than 30), there will be an increased number of women discharged home who will need instruction in self-administration of LMWH.

Risk assessment

See the section 'Risk assessment' at beginning of this chapter for a full discussion on the midwives' role in risk assessment and prophylaxis pre-conception, at booking, when admitted and during and post delivery. The need for hospitalisation will increase the risk of thromboembolism and timely education about leg exercises, regular fluid intake and correct sitting position may be beneficial in addition to recommended prophylaxis measures.

Clinical assessment for signs and symptoms of VTE

The midwife may examine the woman's legs during each clinical assessment both in the antenatal period and during postnatal examination noting the size, colour and any temperature difference between the limbs. Homan's sign can be used, but it is more important for the midwife to listen to the woman when she is describing symptoms and put these in context. Any signs and symptoms of DVT or possible minor or major PE should be referred immediately to medical staff, and diagnosis actively pursued.

General preventative advice

As pregnancy itself increases a woman's risk of developing a DVT, midwives should give information to all pregnant women on ways to prevent venous stasis and promote venous return. Regular exercise such as walking and drinking adequate fluids will help. Pregnant women should avoid sitting with their legs crossed or standing for prolonged periods of time and may find it helpful to put their legs up when sitting down. They should avoid long car journeys without stopping to move around. If in a train or plane, they should walk around and do leg exercises, including ankle flexion and extension. Wearing support stockings will not only prevent feelings of tiredness and strain on the legs but may also work to prevent varicose veins. Some women will be advised to wear TED stockings. Pregnant women should avoid wearing constrictive garments around their legs and pelvic area.

Conclusion

Prevention and detection of thromboembolism in pregnancy is essential in preventing deaths from PE. Risk assessment tools have recently been developed to aid midwives and doctors in identifying women at risk. Midwives need to be alert to the signs and symptoms of DVT, particularly in those with additional risk factors, and make appropriate referral. Prevention of thromboembolism in pregnancy includes the use of effective prophylactic measures and client education.

As in any emergency situation, if a woman collapses with a major PE, the midwife must summon senior medical staff and implement appropriate resuscitation procedures immediately.

References

1 Lewis G, editor. (2007) The Confidential Enquiry into Maternal and Child Health (CEMACH). *Saving Mothers' Lives: Reviewing Maternal Deaths to Make Motherhood Safer 2003–2005. The seventh report on Confidential Enquiries into Maternal Deaths in the UK.* London: CEMACH.

2 Rodger M, Rosene-Montella K, Barbour L. (2008) Acute thromboembolic disease. In: Rosene-Montella, K, Keely E, Barbour L, *et al.*, editors. *Medical Care of the Pregnant Patient.* 2nd ed. Philadelphia: ACP Press, pp. 426–44.

3 Lyons G, Kocarev M. (2007) Thromboembolism. In: Dob D, Cooper G, Holdcroft A, editors. *Crises in Childbirth: why mothers survive.* Oxford: Radcliffe. pp. 147–58.

4 Bourjeily G, Paidas M, Khalil H, *et al.* (2010) Pulmonary embolism in pregnancy. *Lancet.* **375**: 500–12.

5 Jacobsen AF, Skjeldestad FE, Sandset PM. (2008) Incidence and risk patterns of venous thromboembolism in pregnancy and puerperium: a register-based case-control study. *Am J Obstet Gynecol.* **198**(2): 233.e1–e7.

6 Pomp ER, Lenselink AM, Rosendaal FR, Doggen CJ. (2008) Pregnancy and postpartum period and prothrombotic defects: risk of venous thrombosis in the MEGA study. *J Thromb Haemost.* **6**: 632–7.

7 Blanco-Molina A, Trujillo-Santos J, Criado J, *et al.* (2007) Venous thromboembolism during pregnancy or postpartum: findings from the RIETE Registry. *J Thromb Haemost.* **97**(2): 186–90.

8 James AH. (2008) Thromboembolism in pregnancy: recurrence risks, prevention and management. *Curr Opin Obstet Gynecol.* **20**: 550–6.

9 Rosenberg VA, Lockwood CJ. (2007) Thromboembolism in pregnancy. *Obstet Gynecol Clin North Am.* **34**(3): 481–500, xi.

10 Knight M, on behalf of UKOSS. (2008) Antenatal pulmonary embolism: risk factors, management and outcomes. *Br J Obstet Gynaecol.* **115**: 453–61.

11 Greer IA, Thomson AJ. (2001) Management of venous thromboembolism in pregnancy. *Best Pract Res Clin Obstet Gynaecol.* **15**(4): 583–603.

12 Girling J. (2004) Thromboembolism and thrombophilia. *Curr Obstet Gynaecol.* **14**(1): 11–22.

13 Royal College of Obstetricians and Gynaecologists (RCOG). (1995) *RCOG Working Party on Prophylaxis against Thromboembolism in Gynaecology and Obstetrics.* London: RCOG.

14 Lewis G, Drife J. (2001) *Why Mothers Die 1997–1999. The fifth report of the*

Confidential Enquiries into Maternal Deaths in the UK. London: RCOG Press.

15 Royal College of Obstetricians and Gynaecologists (RCOG). (2004) *Green-top Guideline No. 37: thromboprophylaxis during pregnancy, labour and after vaginal delivery.* London: RCOG.

16 Lewis G. (2004) *Why Mothers Die 2000–2002. The sixth report of the Confidential Enquiries into Maternal Deaths in the UK.* London: RCOG Press.

17 Whapshott HC. (2007) Antenatal assessment for risk of venous thromboembolism. *Br J Midwif.* **15**(9): 545–9.

18 Royal College of Obstetricians and Gynaecologists (RCOG). (2009) *Green-top Guideline No. 37: reducing the risk of thrombosis and embolism during pregnancy and the puerperium.* London: RCOG.

19 Bates SM, Greer IA, Pabinger I, Sofaer S, Hirsh J. (2008) Venous thromboembolism, thrombophilia, antithrombotic therapy, and pregnancy: American College of Chest Physicians Evidence Based Clinical Practice Guidelines (8th edition). *Chest.* **133**(Suppl. 6): S844–6.

20 Lim W, Elkelboom JW, Ginsberg JS. (2007) Inherited thrombophilia and pregnancy associated venous thromboembolism. *BMJ.* **334**: 1053–4.

21 James AH, Jamison MG, Brancazio LR, Myers ER. (2006) Venous thromboembolism during pregnancy and the postpartum period: incidence, risk factors, and mortality. *Am J Obstet Gynecol.* **194**(5): 1311–15.

22 Kuperminic MJ. (2003) Thrombophilia and pregnancy. *Reprod Biol Endocrinol.* **14**(1): 111.

23 Robertson L, Greer IA. (2005) Thromboembolism in pregnancy. *Curr Opin Obstet Gynecol.* **17**: 113–16.

24 Calderwood CJ. (2006) Thromboembolism and thrombophilia in pregnancy. *Curr Obstet Gynaecol.* **16**: 321–6.

25 Khare M, Nelson-Piercy C. (2003) Acquired thrombophilias and pregnancy.

Best Pract Res Clin Obstet Gynaecol. **17**(3): 491–507.

26 Wu O, Greer IA. (2007) Is screening for thrombophilia cost-effective? *Curr Opin Haematol.* **14**: 500–3.

27 Robertson L, Wu O, Greer IA. (2004) Thrombophilia and adverse pregnancy outcome. *Curr Opin Obstet Gynecol.* **16**: 453–8.

28 Sebire N, Jolly M, Harris J, *et al.* (2001) Maternal obesity and pregnancy outcome: a study of 287,213 pregnancies in London. *Int J Obes.* **25**: 1175–82.

29 Robinson S, Yu C (2007) The epidemiology of obesity and pregnancy complications. In: Baker P, Balen A, Poston L, *et al.*, editors. *Obesity and Reproductive Health.* London: RCOG Press. pp. 113–26.

30 Lidegaard O, Edstrom B, Kreiner S. (2002) Oral contraceptives and venous thromboembolism: a five year national case-control study. *Contraception.* **65**: 187–96.

31 van Walraven C, Mamdani M, Cohn A, *et al.* (2003) Risk of subsequent thromboembolism for patients with pre-eclampsia. *BMJ.* **326**(12): 791–2.

32 Kovacevich GJ, Gaich SA, Lavin JP, *et al.* (2000). The prevalence of thromboembolic events among women with extended bedrest prescribed as part of the treatment for premature labor or preterm premature rupture of membranes. *Am J Obstet Gynecol.* **182**: 1089–92.

33 Royal College of Obstetricians and Gynaecologists (RCOG). (2008) *Air Travel and Pregnancy: Scientific Advisory Committee Opinion Paper No 1.* London: RCOG Press.

34 Lewis G, Drife J. (1998) *Why Mothers' Die. Report on the Confidential Enquiry into Maternal Deaths in the UK 1994–1996.* London: Department of Health.

35 Jain S, Eedarapalli P, Jamjute P, Sawdy R. (2006) Symphysis pubis dysfunction: a practical approach to management. *The Obstetrician & Gynaecologist.* **8**(3): 153–8.

36 Walker L, Lamont S. (2008) Graduated compression stockings to prevent deep vein thrombosis. *Nurs Stand.* **22**(40): 35–9.

37 Jamieson R, Calderwood CJ, Greer

IA. (2007) The effect of graduated compression stockings on blood velocity in the deep venous system of the lower limb in the postnatal period. *BJOG*. **114**: 1292–4.

38 Casele H, Grobman WA. (2006) Cost-effectiveness of thromboprophylaxis with intermittent pneumatic compression at cesarean delivery. *Obstet Gynecol*. **108**(3/1): 535–40.

39 Phillips S, Gallagher M, Buchan H. (2008) Use graduated compression stockings postoperatively to prevent deep vein thrombosis. *BMJ*. **336**: 943–4.

40 Brady D, Raingruber B, Peterson J, Varnau W, Denman J, *et al.* (2007) The use of knee-length versus thigh-length compression stockings and sequential compression devices. *Crit Care Nurs Q*. **30**(3): 255–62.

41 Gray G, Ash A. (2006) A survey of pregnant women on the use of graduated elastic compression stockings on the antenatal ward. *J Obstet Gynaecol*. **26**(5): 424–8.

42 Welch E. (2006) The assessment and management of venous thromboembolism. *Nurs Stand*. **20**(28): 58–64.

43 Clark P. (2008) Maternal venous thrombosis. *Eur J Obstet Gynecol Reprod Biol*. **139**(1): 3–10.

44 Farquharson RG, Greaves M. (2006) Thromboembolic disease. In: James DK, Gonik, Steer P, editors. *High Risk Pregnancy: management options*. 3rd ed. Philadelphia: Saunders Elsevier. pp. 938–48.

45 To MS, Hunt BJ, Nelson-Piercy C. (2008) A negative D-dimer does not exclude venous thromboembolism (VTE) in pregnancy. *J Obstet Gynaecol*. **28**(2): 222–40.

46 Royal College of Obstetricians and Gynaecologists (RCOG). (2007) *Green-top Guideline No. 28: thromboembolic disease in pregnancy and the puerperium: acute management*. London: RCOG Press.

47 Royal College of Obstetrics and Gynaecology (RCOG). (2008) Venous thrombosis in pregnancy and after birth. Information for you. Available at: www.rcog.org.uk/files/rcog-corp/uploaded-files/PIVenousThrombosis2007.pdf (accessed 23 February 2010).

48 Ahearn G, Hadjiliadis M, Govert J, *et al.* (2002) Massive pulmonary embolism during pregnancy successfully treated with recombinant tissue plasminogen activator. *Arch Intern Med*. **162**: 1221–7.

49 Kawamata K, Chiba Y, Tanaka R, *et al.* (2005) Experience of temporary inferior vena cava filters inserted in the perinatal period to prevent pulmonary embolism in pregnant women with deep vein thrombosis. *J Vasc Surg*. **41**: 652–6.

50 Greer IA, Nelson-Piercy C. (2005) Low molecular-weight heparins for thromboprophylaxis and treatment of venous thromboembolism in pregnancy: a systematic review of safety and efficacy. *Blood*. **106**(2): 401–7.

51 Quinlan D, McQuillan A, Eikelboom J. (2004) Low-molecular-weight heparin compared with intravenous unfractionated heparin for treatment of pulmonary embolism: a meta-analysis of randomized, controlled trials. *Ann Intern Med*. **140**: 175–83.

52 Jilma B, Kamath S, Lip GY. (2003) Antithrombotic therapy in special circumstances. I – pregnancy and cancer. *BMJ*. **4**(326/7379): 37–40.

53 Blann, A. (2006) *Routine Blood Tests Explained*. Oxford: M&K Publishing. pp. 27–34.

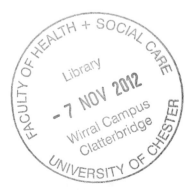

CHAPTER 4

Pre-eclampsia and eclampsia

Maureen Boyle and Sandra McDonald

Pre-eclampsia

Pre-eclampsia may be described as an unpredictable and progressive condition with the potential to cause multi-organ dysfunction and failure that can be detrimental to the woman's health and that of her fetus. There is a suggestion that there may even be two syndromes associated with pre-eclampsia, a maternal syndrome (hypertension and proteinuria with or without multi-organ involvement) and a fetal syndrome (intrauterine growth restriction and other fetal compromise).[1] In the UK it is suggested that about 3%–5% of pregnancies may be affected by pre-eclampsia,[2] while pre-eclampsia and eclampsia are the second most common direct cause of maternal mortality[3]. In other developed countries pre-eclampsia is also considered a major cause of maternal mortality (15%–20%), and in other parts of the world with limited antenatal care, the numbers are much higher.[1] Although fatalities associated with pre-eclampsia in the UK are relatively low in comparison, any fetal death causes anguish and a maternal death is an unimaginable tragedy for the family

concerned, and is possibly an indicator of failure in the care system.

The widespread availability of antenatal care in the UK has given rise to increased surveillance and detection of pre-eclampsia. The results have been timely intervention, improvement in women's care and managed delivery of the baby, all of which have led to reduction in the number of women seen with severe pre-eclampsia, eclampsia and the accompanying complications involving the liver, lungs and brain.[3-5] Nevertheless, *Confidential Enquiries into Maternal Deaths* have identified substandard care in a significant number of cases in the UK.[3] However, pre-eclampsia is a particularly difficult condition, and all experienced midwives will recall women with severe symptoms who made an uncomplicated recovery, as well as women with relatively mild symptoms who suffered a tragic outcome; all emphasising that pre-eclampsia with its high degree of unpredictability is a particular challenge for health professionals.

Midwives at the forefront of maternity care delivery are ideally placed for primary surveillance and early detection of pre-eclampsia. This may prevent an emergency situation occurring and is thus instrumental to the outcome of any individual pregnancy.

While it is not within the remit of this chapter to provide a thorough exposé of the pathophysiology of pre-eclampsia, it is necessary to look at the ways in which the disease process affects the activities of the midwife in the screening process. The initial difficulty lies in definition and the conflicting terminologies used to describe this medical condition. All practitioners will be familiar with what has become the standard description of pre-eclampsia, i.e. 'the occurrence of hypertension and proteinuria (and oedema) after 20 weeks' gestation in a previously normotensive woman'.[6] However, there are uncertainties and dilemmas related to this definition, such as, for example, the exact blood pressure measurements that are to be used in defining hypertension, the quantitative value of proteinuria measured and the fact that oedema is a physiologically normal clinical event in the latter part of pregnancy. Further subdivisions are made as to whether the condition should be defined as mild or severe based on the proffered criteria. Some women with relatively high blood pressures developed during pregnancy may not seem to have an apparently progressive disease and their babies continue to thrive. Others may present with proteinuria (in which contaminant and infection has been excluded), have pronounced clinical oedema and indications of intrauterine growth restriction of the fetus, but still have normal blood pressure. An even smaller number will show no traditionally acceptable evidence of pre-eclampsia, but present with a non-specific history of feeling unwell and only biochemical investigations reveal the true nature of the disease.

Although it is acknowledged that pre-eclampsia is a very unpredictable disease and may occur in those with no predisposing factors, it may be useful to consider those who have been suggested as being at increased risk of developing this condition (*see* Box 4.1).

> **BOX 4.1** Risk factors for pre-eclampsia[1,6,7]
> - Primigravida
> - Pre-eclampsia in a previous pregnancy
> - >10 years since the last pregnancy
> - Extremes of maternal age
> - Second or subsequent pregnancy with a new partner
> - History of pre-eclampsia in mother or sister
> - Women with partners who previously fathered a pre-eclamptic pregnancy
> - Multiple pregnancy
> - Diastolic blood pressure >80 mmHg at booking
> - Proteinuria at booking
> - History of essential hypertension before pregnancy
> - Women with pre-existing medical conditions, e.g. diabetics or renal disease
> - BMI >35 at booking
> - A pregnancy involving donor material
> - Antiphospholipid antibodies
> - Hydrops fetalis, hydatidiform mole or polyhydramnios.

Pathophysiology

The aetiology of pre-eclampsia remains unknown, but understanding of the pathogenesis has been advanced in recent years by laboratory work and evidence is becoming increasingly available that the various theories presented have some common features.[1] In a healthy pregnancy uncomplicated by pre-eclampsia, trophoblastic cells invade the maternal uterine arteries at both the decidual and myometrial level, resulting in erosion of the muscle layer and enlargement of the lumen. Additionally, there is increased synthesis of prostacyclin, nitric oxide and thromboxane A_2, which create a change in homeostatic balance and tendency to vasodilatation of the uterine arteries. This alteration in function results in lowered resistance in the arteries, absence of maternal vasomotor control and a massive increase in blood supply to the placenta to meet the demands of the developing fetus.[8] The associated changes account for the transient lowering of maternal blood pressure seen in early pregnancy, which is then compensated for by the physiologic increase in circulating volume.

The changes seen in pre-eclampsia appear to be caused by a complex interplay of abnormal genetic, immunological and placental factors.[9] The early changes in the way the placenta embeds in the uterus is considered to be significant, in that trophoblastic invasion of the placental bed spiral arteries is confined to the decidual level. As a result of this arrested trophoblastic invasion, adrenergic nerve supplies to the uterine spiral arteries are not disrupted, systemic vascular resistance remains high and placental perfusion is poor. The resultant effect is tissue hypoxia, which is believed to cause liberation of substances that are toxic to endothelial cells.[1,10] It has been suggested that this involves an inflammatory response.[1] Enhanced contraction of damaged blood vessels facilitates aggregation of platelets at the site of injury. Production of oxygen free radicals, failure of haemodilution, reduced glomerular filtration and poor renal reabsorption all combine to give the presentation seen in pre-eclampsia.

Blood pressure

Practitioners are cautioned that any rise in blood pressure occurring after 20 weeks' gestation in a previously normotensive woman should be cause for concern, as this may be the first indicator of a progressive disorder. However, while not underestimating the significance of a rise in blood pressure in combination with other clinical features, it has been suggested that in isolation such a rise may have little effect on the pregnancy, especially in the last trimester.[5]

A diastolic blood pressure recording of 90 mmHg has long been accepted as one sign of pre-eclampsia, but in isolation it may not necessarily be unsafe if it plateaus at this level. However, a progressive rise is associated with an increase in maternal and neonatal morbidity and mortality.[5] Although traditionally the diastolic reading has always been seen as the most important, it has recently been identified that equal attention should be paid to the systolic reading,[3,11] and treatment guidelines are suggested for hypertension defined as 140/90 and severe hypertension with blood pressures of 160/110 or greater.[3,11]

The practising midwife can combine the above information and her knowledge of physiology when screening women for pre-eclampsia. Equally, she needs to be aware of other factors such as any recent physical activity undertaken, the emotions of the woman and the time of day the blood pressure is recorded, as all of these may have an impact upon the accuracy of her observation. *The Report on Confidential Enquiries into Maternal Deaths* over the past two trienniums[3,12] has warned against exclusive reliance on automated blood pressure recording systems. While useful for establishing a trend over several readings,[13] conventional mercury sphygmomanometers remain the instrument of choice in order to prevent underestimation of the blood pressure. However, since in many units this equipment is no longer available, care must be taken to check the automated reading against another validated device if concerned.[11]

Blood pressure evaluation is such a routine part of midwifery practice it would be easy to become complacent. However, when considered objectively, numerous factors such as the woman's personal fluctuations, the possibilities of 'white coat syndrome', work stress, less than perfect auditory acuity and a noisy working environment all make blood pressure recording anything but straightforward or simple. However, accuracy of assessment as part of professional midwifery practice is vital for women's well-being.[14]

Proteinuria

No dispute seems to exist in the literature as to the importance of proteinuria in the diagnosis of pre-eclampsia, and the fact that increasing levels of proteinuria are associated with adverse maternal and fetal outcomes,[15] but what is debatable is the amount of protein considered significant. The reagent strips ('dipsticks') commonly used in clinical practice should be considered a guide only to the presence of protein in the urine and not be accepted as an accurate quantification

of protein excretion.[16] It should also be ensured that manufacturer's instructions concerning care of dipsticks (such as dating the opening of bottles and replacing lids after use) are followed to ensure accuracy is optimal.

When any amount of protein is detected, a clean-caught mid-stream sample of urine should be tested to exclude the possibility of contamination. If protein is still detectable, the sample should be sent to the laboratory for exclusion of infection and a 24-hour urine collection should be obtained for protein assessment. It has been suggested that more than 0.3 g in a 24-hour collection is significant. A urine specimen may be sent for a laboratory urinary spot protein:creatinine ratio (PCR) to assess first whether a 24-hour urinary collection is necessary.[17]

Practitioners are reminded that the quantity of protein present in urine samples may not be indicative of renal damage, but instead may be a reflection of capillary leakage and more accurately a projection of the development of generalised oedema. Where protein loss is significant, the possibility of pulmonary and cerebral oedema as complications of pre-eclampsia is considerable.

Serology

While the worsening of the combination of two of the cardinal signs, proteinuria and hypertension, are acceptable as reasonable predictors of increasingly severe pre-eclampsia, it is as well to remember that women with blood pressures within the normal range, or in whom proteinuria was absent, have had eclamptic fits. The obvious presence of a single finding should prompt investigations for others by measuring known biochemical markers (*see* Box 4.2 for an example of blood routinely taken for PET screening). When bloods are taken for a PET screening, if the results are within the normal range, they can act as a baseline for future tests. A rising level, even if the results are still within the normal range, should act as a warning sign, and these blood results should be recorded in a way that any trend is easily identifiable.

BOX 4.2 PET Screening

While many tests may be carried out, of particular importance are:

Full blood count:
- haemoglobin
- platelets.

Renal function tests ~ urine:
- creatinine clearance
- total urinary protein.

Renal function tests ~ blood:
- creatinine
- uric acid (urates)
- urea.

Liver function tests:
- AST (aspartate aminotransferase)
- ALT (alanine aminotransferase)
- Alkaline phosphatase
- Total albumin.

Clotting studies may also be carried out.

While the midwife may initiate many of the early biochemical and haematological investigations and is eminently able to interpret findings, she must remember the scope of her clinical practice and always act in accordance with the Midwives Rules and Standards,[18] referring the woman to a registered medical practitioner when there are signs of deviation from normal.

Full blood count

FBC is a valuable assessment in pre-eclampsia as much information can be gained. Normal pregnancy results in physiological haemodilution and lower levels of erythrocytes in a specified volume of blood, although their life span is not affected. In pre-eclampsia the reduction in intravascular volume causes a rise in haematocrit and polycythaemia, while erythrocytes are damaged by the friction of their forced passage within the damaged endothelial lining of blood vessels. Repeated damage significantly reduces the life expectancy of erythrocytes, leading to increased haemolysis and anaemia.

Mild thrombocytopaenia, the cause of which is unknown, has long been identified as an uncomplicated finding in normal pregnancy; but when present in pre-eclampsia the platelet levels should be closely and regularly monitored. Reduction in platelets is thought to be related to a shorter life span and aggregation at the site of endothelial vascular damage, secondary to the hypertensive state, but acute presentation (indicated by a fall of 20%–30% from the baseline measurement in early pregnancy) is associated with severe pre-eclampsia and HELLP syndrome.

Renal function tests

In pregnancy urea and creatinine clearance is high, but blood levels at the upper end of the range may be suggestive of impaired renal clearance. A rise in serum uric acid production is secondary to tissue ischaemia and increasing levels may be reflective of impaired renal clearance, renal medullary ischaemia and tubular damage[16] and these findings may be the only clinical indicators of the seriousness of pre-eclampsia. The importance of this information is that a rise in serum uric acid can be detected before proteinuria becomes evident.

Leakage of albumin through the kidneys is a positive indication of glomerular endothelial damage, the consequences of which are lowering of serum albumin levels and leakage of fluid into the extra cellular space, while a marked rise in serum creatinine is indicative of severe renal impairment.

Liver function tests

Development of epigastric or right upper quadrant pain is indicative of liver involvement. Damage to the endothelial lining of blood vessels in the liver results in leakage of plasma and causes an increase in size and overstretching of the fibrous capsule. In addition, blood vessels may rupture and haematoma may form in the sub-capsular region, increasing the pressure on the liver peritoneum with referred pain.

There is a need for the midwife to be aware of differential causes of abdominal pain; for example, acute fatty liver disease. This dangerous condition of unknown origin is similar in presentation to pre-eclampsia, with symptoms of headache, abdominal pain, vomiting and reduced urinary output, and can complicate its diagnosis.

Raised levels of liver enzymes such as alanine aminotransferase, aspartate aminotransferase and bilirubin, in combination with placental alkaline phosphatase, are indicators of a significant level of liver cell damage and the development of HELLP syndrome.

Therapy for reducing hypertension

The aim of drug therapy is to prevent the development of very severe hypertension and so avert the development of seizure, and reduce the risks of cerebrovascular accidents, emergency and preterm delivery of the baby, as well as the accompanying perinatal risks. However, treatment is dependent on the individual woman's condition and cannot be successfully predicted, so close observation is always necessary.

An array of hypotensive treatments have been used to minimise the risk of cerebral damage associated with pre-eclampsia, but it must be borne in mind that these are not cures as they do not arrest the disease progression. Antihypertensives are considered vital when a blood pressure is >160/110[11] but medication is often commenced before this level is reached. A brief description of the mode of action of some of the more common drugs used to manage pre-eclampsia follows.

Angiotensin converting enzyme (ACE) inhibitors: e.g. captopril, enalapril

ACE inhibitors are powerful hypotensive agents that reduce blood pressure by stimulating vasodilation and inhibiting the enzyme necessary for converting angiotensin I to angiotensin II (the latter being a powerful vasoconstrictor). While highly effective for controlling hypertension in non-pregnant individuals or after delivery, they have limited success in pregnancy and are no longer used in pregnancy as an association with fetal skeletal defects has been suggested.

Central alpha-II agonist: e.g. methyldopa

This is a centrally acting hypotensive drug used in the first line of management in pregnancy. It is an alpha-II agonist acting directly on the brainstem to create vasodilation and lowering of the blood pressure without adverse changes in heart rate, cardiac output, renal perfusion or uteroplacental blood flow. Lowering of the blood pressures is slow, thus where rapid onset of hypotension is desired an alternative drug is preferable.

Alpha and beta sympathetic blocking agents: e.g. labetalol, metoprolol, atenolol

This group of peripheral-acting sympatholytic drugs includes alpha, beta and combined alpha + beta sympathetic blocking agents. They act on blood vessels by altering the baroreceptor sympathetic reflex response of nerves to adrenergic vasoconstrictors such as prostaglandins. The resultant effects are maintained vascular relaxation, lowered peripheral resistance and reduced cardiac output, thus lowering the blood pressure. Labetalol is often given in severe pre-eclampsia as an intravenous infusion.

Arteriolar dilator: e.g. hydralazine

Hydralazine is usually reserved for use in cases of very high blood pressure. Given intravenously, it acts directly on the smooth muscles of the arterial wall to bring about vasodilation in 10 to 20 minutes with the hypotensive effect lasting six to eight hours. Side-effects are headaches, nausea and vomiting (signs which mimic impending eclampsia) and a possible link to thrombocytopaenia in the neonate has been reported. Care needs to be taken to avoid a very rapid drop in blood pressure in a pregnant woman, which could lead to reduced placental perfusion and fetal distress.

Calcium channel blockers: e.g. nifedipine (Adalat®)

This drug belongs to the group of calcium antagonists and has increasingly been used in pre-eclampsia as the second line in hypertensive management where early treatment with methyldopa has failed to keep maternal blood pressure below the danger level. The effect of the drug is rapid. The sublingual route is not normally used in pregnancy, because mucosal absorption is unpredictable.[19] It works by preventing transfer of calcium ions from extracellular space and inhibits uptake by smooth muscle cells. Vascular muscle response and reflex excitation contractility is reduced and relaxation is achieved, peripheral resistance is lowered and blood vessels dilate and blood pressure falls.

Magnesium sulphate

Magnesium sulphate is recommended as a first-line treatment of eclampsia and to prevent eclampsia in those at high risk. Although its primary function is as an anticonvulsive, it also has a strong hypotensive effect, and further antihypertensive medication may not be necessary (*see* later in this chapter for midwifery care when a woman is receiving a magnesium sulphate infusion).

In the past specific warning has been given when administering magnesium sulphate where nifedipine has previously been taken, as this combination may increase the plasma concentration and thus the potency of the drug,[19] although this no longer appears problematic.[20] However, it is not recommended that nifedipine is taken with grapefruit or grapefruit juice, as this may potentiate the hypotensive effect.

The choice of which drug is used in practice is probably related to familiarity as this does instil confidence, a factor essential to the prompt and successful management of the woman's condition. The midwife needs to ensure she knows the protocol and policies of her workplace, as these will be different from unit to unit.

HELLP syndrome

HELLP (Haemolysis, Elevated Liver enzymes and Low Platelets) syndrome is a serious complication usually associated with pre-eclampsia but in which many women do not develop significant hypertension or proteinuria.[21] Its development is a clear indication for close surveillance. Diagnosis is based on a combination of laboratory findings, clinical signs and symptoms (*see* Box 4.3), although these may vary significantly. It has been suggested that 20% of women had not been diagnosed with pre-eclampsia before delivery and one-third of women with HELLP syndrome will be diagnosed postnatally.[21]

The full blood count is an invaluable screening tool for HELLP, as evidence of anaemia may indicate excessive breakdown of red cells, one of the early features. Irrespective of the cause of anaemia, haemolysis or iron deficiency, it must be borne in mind that its presence will increase the cardiac workload and thus exacerbate hypertension. Alternatively, a haemoglobin level which is high for pregnancy may be an indicator of haemoconcentration with reduced intravascular volume and secondary to marked oedema.

The life span of platelets in pre-eclampsia can be reduced by approximately 50% (from nine to five days); additionally, there is an increased level of activation and enhanced adhesion capacity at the site of endothelial cell damage. The combined

---

BOX 4.3 HELLP syndrome

Possible signs and symptoms
- Right upper quadrant pain (and often with a positive liver recoil test)
- Epigastric pain
- Nausea and vomiting
- Malaise
- Generalised oedema
- Fatigue
- Headache
- Gastrointestinal bleed
- Hypertension
- Proteinuria
- Reduced urine output.

Possible laboratory findings
- Haemolysis
- Anaemia
- Low platelet count (<100 × 10^9/l)
- Elevated liver enzymes:
  - alanine aminotransferase
  - aspartate aminotransferase
  - gamma glutamyltransferase
- Elevated levels of bilirubin.

---

effects of these actions lead to a continuing fall in platelet count and development of thrombocytopaenia, while the multisystem failure in HELLP is associated with changes in renal and hepatic function.

Reduced circulatory volume, ischaemia, renal tubular necrosis and reduced renal clearance lead to a rise in the levels of urea, creatinine and serum urate which are indicators of marked maternal and fetal compromise. Infarctions and oedema occurring in the liver will impair its capacity to maintain adequate metabolic activities such as synthesis of clotting factors, while increase in liver size may lead to capsular rupture, triggering a combined medical, surgical and obstetric emergency.

Management of HELLP syndrome

Hospitalisation is required to enable more intense monitoring of the maternal and fetal condition with the aim of stabilisation and expediting the birth (*see* Box 4.4). The time available for measures to be initiated is dictated by the woman's condition, fetal maturity and the clinical facilities available for safe delivery and management of a possible preterm infant. For some women the condition may develop rapidly and before a stage where fetal viability is a possibility, while for others the progression of disease may be more gradual.

BOX 4.4 Optimal management of HELLP syndrome

- Timely diagnosis and ongoing accurate assessment of the severity
- Control of blood pressure if necessary
- Prevention of seizure
- Management of fluid and electrolytes balance
- Assessment and monitoring of fetal condition
- Planning and management of delivery
- Judicious care to manage the potential for haemorrhage
- Maximum supportive care to enhance the baby's survival
- High dependency or intensive care for the woman postpartum, with awareness of the continued risk of multiple organ failure
- Counselling about future pregnancies.

Where timing permits, in that the woman's condition does not present an immediate threat, strategies may be implemented to assess fetal well-being and improve survival rates. This may include biophysical assessment by ultrasound to determine the degree of hypoxaemia and fetal reserve, administration of corticosteroids to accelerate fetal lung maturity in prematurity and continual assessing of fetal well-being by cardiotocography. The woman's condition should also be closely observed for detection of the onset of labour or rapid disease progression, indicated by deterioration in her blood results or increasing severity of physical signs and symptoms.

Fulminating pre-eclampsia

Fulminating pre-eclampsia is a severe medical condition which should be thought of as an emergency. It is essentially a fractional window of opportunity, the duration of which cannot be predicted with any certainty, when timely intervention and appropriate treatment may prevent a seizure. Essentially, there are two possible courses of action related to management, either immediate delivery where risk to the woman would be greater if the pregnancy was continued or prolongation of the pregnancy within a controlled environment once her condition has been stabilised. The latter course will permit administration of corticosteroids to assist fetal lung maturity and benefit the baby which will be born early. While an active search and treat programme is the goal of antenatal care, it offers no guarantee against development of severe pre-eclampsia or eclampsia and it is important that midwifery practitioners know that convulsion may be the first and only indication of an underlying pathological process.

Changes associated with a worsening condition do not necessarily follow a logical, sequential or linear progression, nor are seizures predictable.[22] Some women may have a very severe presentation of pre-eclampsia where the practitioner expects the condition to culminate in convulsion, yet this does not happen. Therefore it is imperative that midwives remain watchful for new developments or subtle changes discernible through close physical observation and changes in levels of biochemical tests, and not let reassuring observations or test results diminish attentiveness or create a false sense of security. *See* Box 4.5 for signs and symptoms of fulminating pre-eclampsia.

BOX 4.5 Signs and symptoms of fulminating pre-eclampsia

- Continuing rise in blood pressure
- Increasing proteinuria
- Oliguria
- Development of epigastric pain
- Nausea and vomiting
- Liver tenderness
- Severe headache
- Visual field disturbance (floaters or diplopia)
- Bleeding tendency (platelet count decreasing and abnormal liver enzymes)
- Hyper-reflexia (brisk tendon reflexes)
- Abnormalities in fetal heart assessment.

Blood pressure

The importance of blood pressure measurement has been introduced previously, but in severe pre-eclampsia observations are made and recorded at intervals of between five and 15 minutes, and closely balanced by administration of medication in accordance with prescribed instructions, often titrated to the mean arterial pressure (MAP) reading.[13] The purpose of this is to ensure an appropriate response that is finely balanced to avert seizure or cerebral vascular accident, yet protects against the occurrence of sudden devastating hypotension that can be detrimental to the woman's cerebral function and fetal well-being.

Renal function

Low levels of serum albumin will result in excessive loss of intravascular volume, impact on the cardiovascular system and be evident as oedema. This is indicated as a rise in haematocrit, polycythaemia, reducing renal perfusion, impaired renal tubular function and poor reabsorption of protein, causing further leakage of fluid into the extra cellular space and resulting in reduced urinary output – a vicious cycle is in motion. The woman should be catheterised, the urine measured hourly (output should be 0.5 ml/kg/hr and should not fall below 30 ml/hr) and tested for the quantity of protein.

Serology

Walker[16] suggests that a falling platelet count could be used as a guide to the timing of delivery, as it is associated with a worsening of the maternal and fetal condition. Adhesion of platelets to damaged endothelial blood vessel walls narrows the lumen, reduces end organ perfusion, exacerbates tissue damage through anoxia and predisposes the woman to development of eclampsia, placental abruption and possible fetal demise.

Care of the woman with fulminating pre-eclampsia

Women admitted with fulminating or severe pre-eclampsia must be closely monitored (*see* Box 4.6) and medicated. One-to-one care, with drugs and equipment for managing an eclamptic fit, monitoring the fetal condition and supporting adequate ventilation and oxygen therapy, is essential. A multidisciplinary approach involving obstetrician and anaesthetist at consultant level, haematologist, paediatrician and appropriately experienced midwife should be involved in the planning and provision of care, and the neonatal intensive care unit should be alerted.

Management of the condition necessitates two aims being pursued simultaneously, namely lowering of the blood pressure and intensive observation of maternal and fetal condition. The first objective requires initiation of therapy to lower the blood pressure to a level where the potential for seizure is reduced, thereby protecting the woman's cerebrovascular circulation and preventing a stroke.[3,11] The second objective involves intense monitoring of maternal and fetal condition for early detection of deterioration (impending seizure, organ failure and pulmonary oedema), the onset of labour and/or evidence of fetal compromise. A level of blood pressure around 140/90 mmHg is thought to be a safe compromise as further reductions may well impair placental perfusion and affect fetal well-being.[23]

Fetal growth scans are usually carried out every two weeks, but other means of fetal assessment, including CTG, liquor volume estimation and umbilical artery Doppler assessment, will be done as frequently as necessary, depending on the individual circumstances.

The midwife must record vital signs (at a frequency determined by individual condition, but perhaps as often as every five minutes), with particular attention being paid to blood pressure, oxygen saturation readings and level of consciousness. Medication being used for control of blood pressure should be administered as prescribed, and intake and output levels scrupulously maintained. This will usually involve fluid restriction and hourly urine measurement until the woman is delivered, and/or her medical state is deemed controlled. Central venous pressure and arterial line monitoring may be used and their readings should be regularly recorded. The urine should be tested frequently and the amount of protein quantified. Continuous monitoring of the fetal heart rate pattern is usual.

Nil-by-mouth is usual and intravenous access is essential. Hartmann's solution may be used with strict control of the rate of infusion to reduce the risk of pulmonary oedema and cardiac failure. As a very fine balance between intake and output is required, this may be best achieved by monitoring of the CVP. All unit policies for pre-eclampsia care will contain a section regarding fluid restriction, and midwives will need to remember that bolus drug infusions and oral intake should be included in the 'allowed' amount of fluid.

The importance of meticulous evaluation and recording of input and output cannot be over-emphasised. The Confidential Enquiry into Maternal Deaths[3] credits better fluid management with the recent lack of deaths from pulmonary causes in women with pre-eclampsia.

Clinical biochemical features of full blood count, electrolytes, uric acid, liver enzymes, fibrinogen, platelets, clotting studies and blood urea nitrogen (BUN) should be assessed every four hours or daily as the woman's condition dictates.

If the woman's condition stabilises

sufficiently to enable labour to be induced, an epidural analgesia is often selected where the clotting studies are satisfactory. This method of pain relief offers the additional benefits of lowering blood pressure, elimination of painful stimuli that may trigger convulsion and avoids the possibility of anaesthetic complications which may accompany general anaesthesia and exacerbate pulmonary oedema. It is therefore the preference for caesarean section but requires particular caution, as the pre-epidural fluid load may be sufficient to alter the stable balance previously attained.

There is a 1:200 risk of eclampsia where the woman has had pre-eclampsia, if any difficulty is encountered in achieving control of the blood pressure, or there

---

BOX 4.6 Midwifery care of the woman with fulminating pre-eclampsia

- Monitor vital signs, particularly blood pressure and saturations.
- Administer drugs and assess effect on blood pressure.
- Monitor and record total fluid input and urinary output (and level of proteinuria).
- Monitor fetal condition and assess for onset of labour.
- Obtain blood samples as necessary and monitor results for changes reflecting deterioration.
- Assess for symptoms of worsening condition.
- Maintain a quiet, calm atmosphere.
- Provide psychological care for the woman and her family.
- Any significant changes in the woman's condition must be notified to the obstetrician and/or anaesthetist.

---

are indications of HELLP syndrome, fulminating pre-eclampsia or fetal distress. Therefore such measures as are necessary to hasten fetal lung maturity must be initiated and delivery must be expedited.[16] Effective measures are needed to prevent convulsion, major organ failure, fetal demise, and reduce the severity of postpartum exacerbation and long-term morbidity. However, once a convulsion has occurred the continuation of the pregnancy cannot be justified.

Eclampsia

Eclampsia is the occurrence of convulsions that are associated with the signs and symptoms of pre-eclampsia. It is a Greek word meaning lightning and often strikes with the same random ferocity and has similarly devastating effects. The seizure that is the key feature of eclampsia is thought to be due to intense vasospasm of the cerebral arteries, oedema secondary to ischaemic damage of vascular endothelium and intravascular clot formation.

An eclamptic fit usually includes three defined phases.

1 *Prodromal*, in which the imminent fit is heralded by possible reports of visual disturbances, muscular twitching, facial congestion, foaming at the mouth and/or deepening loss of consciousness.

2 *Tonic-clonic*, where initially generalised muscular contractions are present and respiration is absent. This is followed by repeated strong jerky irregular muscular activity.

3 *Abatement*, which occurs within 60–90 seconds of onset during which time respiration is re-established and there is gradual return to

consciousness, but perhaps with a confused and agitated state.

It is futile to attempt any action within the short interval of the tonoclonic phase apart from protecting the woman from injury. However, subsequent care should be aimed at damage limitation by placing the woman in the recovery position once the seizure has passed. Suction should be used to clear secretions from the mouth and nasal passage to maintain a clear airway and oxygen should be administered. These immediate measures help to boost the maternal oxygen saturation and improve delivery to the fetus which would have been deprived of oxygen during the tonoclonic phase of the seizure.

Further urgent measures are now imperative to prevent the recurrence of further seizure and optimise maternal and fetal well-being (*see* Box 4.7).

Suggested treatment regime using magnesium sulphate

Various therapies combining hypotensive agents and anticonvulsants have been used in recent times to manage pre-eclampsia and eclampsia, but without any consensus on efficacy. However, recent research studies carried out in the USA and UK comparing treatments of eclampsia concluded that magnesium sulphate was effective both as an anticonvulsant and hypotensive agent, both for the treatment of eclampsia and as a preventative.[25,26]

Magnesium sulphate is usually administered intravenously as a loading dose, followed by a maintenance infusion. As magnesium sulphate is a powerful depressant of neuromuscular transmission, extreme care must be taken to avoid sudden hypotension. Additionally, as this

BOX 4.7 Immediate care of the eclamptic woman

- Summon assistance (anaesthetist and obstetrician)/call for emergency paramedic help if at home – immediate transfer to hospital is necessary.
- Protect from injury during the tonoclonic phase.
- Maintain airway (clear by suctioning if necessary).
- Provide supplementary oxygenation.
- Place woman in the left lateral (recovery) position.
- Obtain intravenous access and monitor fluid balance.
- Treat the convulsion.
- Possibly sedate to prevent hyperstimulation.
- Monitor vital signs.
- Assess fetal well-being (risk of fetal distress from hypoxia or abruption).
- Achieve stability of maternal condition.
- Plan mode of delivery.
- Execute plan without further delay.

drug is excreted via the kidneys, existing damage and impaired renal clearance could result in toxic levels being quickly reached. A maximum blood magnesium level of 4 mmol/l is therapeutic, but around 7 mmol/l is associated with respiratory distress, while levels of around 12 mmol/l can trigger cardiac arrest. The frequency with which serum magnesium levels are measured will depend on urinary output as an indicator of renal function and the presence of positive-screening characteristics are indicative of approaching toxicity levels (*see* Box 4.8).

BOX 4.8 Signs and symptoms of magnesium sulphate toxicity

- Loss of tendon reflexes
- Double vision
- Depressed respiration
- Slurred speech
- Flushing
- Weakness
- Reduced urinary output <0.5 ml/kg/hr
- Drowsiness.

Once the woman's condition has stabilised and the baby has been delivered, the aggressive approach to management needs to be maintained as the risk of eclamptic fits occurring during the first 24 hours of the postpartum period remains.

In addition to the physical care the woman requires, there is the need for psychological support as there may be many questions the woman wishes to have answered. The skills of the midwife as communicator will be essential in providing information that is timely, appropriate, accurate and as comprehensive as possible to assist with the process of adjustment to what has been a life-threatening event. The midwife might also consider informing the woman and her partner about Action on Pre-eclampsia (APEC), an organisation where she may be able to obtain continued support and information at a time when she will find it beneficial (www.apec.org.uk).

References

1 Sibai B, Dekker G, Kupferminc M. (2005) Pre eclampsia. *Lancet*. **365**: 785–99.
2 Action on Pre-eclampsia (APEC). Basic information on pre-eclampsia. www.apec.org.uk/preeclampsiabasics.htm (accessed 22 February 2010).
3 Lewis G, editor. (2007) *The Confidential Enquiry into Maternal and Child Health (CEMACH). Saving Mothers' Lives: reviewing maternal deaths to make motherhood safer – 2003–2005. The Seventh Report on Confidential Enquiries into Maternal Deaths in the United Kingdom*. London: CEMACH.
4 Knight M, UKOSS. (2007) Eclampsia in the United Kingdom 2005. *BJOG*. **114**(9): 1072–8.
5 Duley L, Henderson-Smart DJ. (2000) Drugs for rapid treatment of very high blood pressure in pregnancy. *The Cochrane Library*. (Issue 4). Oxford: Update Software.
6 Milne F, Redman C, Walker J, *et al.* (2005) The pre-eclampsia community guideline (PRECOG): how to screen for and detect onset of pre-eclampsia in the community. *BMJ*. **330**: 567–80.
7 Duckitt K, Harrington D. (2005) Risk factors for pre-eclampsia at antenatal booking: systematic review of controlled studies. *BMJ*. **330**: 565–71.
8 Stables D, Rankin J. (2005) *Physiology in Childbearing: with anatomy and related biosciences*. 2nd ed. Edinburgh: Elsevier.
9 Bothamley J, Boyle M. (2009) *Medical Conditions affecting Pregnancy and Childbirth*. Oxford: Radcliffe Publishing.
10 Powrie R, Rosene-Montella K. (2008) Pre-eclampsia. In: Rosene-Montella K, Keely E, Barbour L, *et al.*, editors. *Medical Care of the Pregnant Patient*. 2nd ed. Philadelphia: ACP Press.
11 Royal College of Obstetricians and Gynaecologists (RCOG). (2006) *The Management of Severe Pre-eclampsia/Eclampsia*. Guideline 10(A), March. London: RCOG Press.
12 Lewis G. (2005) *The Confidential Enquiry into Maternal and Child Health (CEMACH). Why mothers die: reviewing maternal deaths to make motherhood safer – 2000–2002. The Sixth Report on Confidential Enquiries into Maternal Deaths in the United Kingdom*. London: CEMACH.
13 Bothamley J, Boyle M. (2008) How to use automated blood pressure monitoring. *Midwives*. April/May: 19.

14 Reinders L, Mos C, Thorton C, *et al.* (2006) Time poor: rushing decreases the accuracy and reliability of blood pressure measurement technique in pregnancy. *Hypertens Pregnancy.* 25(2): 81–91.

15 Thangaratinam S, Coomarasamy A, O'Mahony F, *et al.* (2009) Estimation of proteinuria as a predictor of complications of pre-eclampsia: a systematic review. *BMC Med.* 7(10): [pmid: 19317889] [doi: 10.1186/1741-7015-7-10].

16 Walker JJ. (2000) Severe pre-eclampsia and eclampsia. *Baillieres Clin Obstet Gynaecol.* 14(1): 57–71.

17 Cote A, Brown M, Lam E, *et al.* (2008) Diagnostic accuracy of urinary spot protein: creatinine ratio for proteinuria in hypertensive pregnant women: systematic review. *BMJ.* 335(7651): 103–6.

18 Nursing and Midwifery Council (NMC). (2004) *Midwifery Rules and Standards.* London: NMC.

19 Churchill D, Beevers DG. (1999) Treatment of hypertensive disorders of pregnancy. In: Churchill D, Beevers DG, editors. *Hypertension in Pregnancy.* London: BMJ Books.

20 Magee L, Miremadi S, Li J, *et al.* (2005) Therapy with both magnesium sulfate and nifedipine does not increase the risk of serious magnesium-related maternal side effects in women with preeclampsia. *Am J Obstet Gynecol.* 193(1): 153–63.

21 Norwitz E, Hsu C, Repke J. (2002) Acute complications of preeclampsia. *Clin Obstet Gynecol.* 45(2): 308–29.

22 Kats VL, Farmer R, Kuller JA. (2000) Pre-eclampsia into eclampsia: towards a new paradigm. *Am J Obstet Gynecol.* 182(6): 1389–96.

23 Chamberlain G, Steer P. (1999) ABC of labour care: labour in special circumstances. *BMJ.* 318(7191): 1124–7.

24 Moodley J, Jjuuko G, Rout C. (2001) Epidural compared with general anaesthetic for caesarean section delivery in conscious women with eclampsia. *Br J Obstet Gynaecol.* 108: 378–82.

25 Williams J, Mozurkewich E, Chilimigras J, Van de Ven C. (2008) Critical care in obstetrics: pregnancy-specific conditions. *Best Pract Res Clin Obstet Gynaecol.* 22(5): 825–46.

26 Duley L, Meher S, Abalos E. (2006) Management of pre-eclampsia. *BMJ.* 332: 463–8.

CHAPTER 5

Antepartum haemorrhage

Hazel Sundle

Introduction

Antepartum haemorrhage (APH) occurs in approximately 2%–5% of all pregnancies and can be defined as bleeding from the genital tract after 24 weeks' gestation and before the birth of the baby. The basis of this definition is in keeping with the current national legal age of viability of the fetus.[2-4] In America this definition is considered from 20 weeks' gestation.[2,3] If the woman is in labour, similar bleeding is called intrapartum haemorrhage (*see* Chapter 10). The types of antepartum haemorrhage can be described as:

- accidental: as in placental abruption
- incidental: from local lesions in the genital tract
- inevitable: as in placenta praevia.

Any bleeding in pregnancy can be very serious and potentially life threatening to the fetus and/or the mother. Third trimester bleeding is still a main cause of perinatal morbidity and mortality. The most common causes of dangerous bleeding in the latter part of pregnancy are placental abruption (abruptio placentae), and placenta praevia. Just over half of the

women who present with an antepartum haemorrhage are found to have one of these two conditions. There is often no firm diagnosis made for the other half, whose bleeding is said to be 'unclassified' or 'bleeding of unknown origin'. However, some of these causes have been noted as being from varicosities, a 'show', genital tract trauma, polyps, tumours, vasa praevia and infections such as cervicitis or vaginitis.[2-4] There is evidence to suggest that women who have experienced antenatal bleeding of unknown origin (ABUO) are at greater risk of preterm delivery and term labour induction. Their neonates are at greater risk for admissions to SCBU, reduced birth weight and raised bilirubin levels.[5]

Vasa praevia, the only fetal cause of APH, occurs when there is a velamentous insertion of the umbilical cord, i.e. the blood vessels run through the membranes, and run across the lower segment of the uterus in front of the presenting part.[1] *See* Chapter 10 for a description of vasa praevia, a possible cause (albeit fetal) of APH.

It is recommended that women presenting with any vaginal bleeding should be followed up carefully antenatally to monitor the bleeding and fetal well-being, as such bleeding is associated with a high perinatal mortality rate.

According to the most recent *Report on Confidential Enquiries into Maternal and Child Health*,[6] there were two maternal deaths due to placental abruption and three due to placenta praevia from 2003 to 2005.

Risk or predisposing factors

- **For abruption:** These include bleeding in the first trimester, pre-eclampsia, hypertension, smoking, drug use such as cocaine, blunt abdominal trauma, external cephalic version (ECV), multiple pregnancy, increasing age and parity, recurrence (i.e. 4%–8%), acute and chronic respiratory diseases, vitamin deficiency.
- **For placenta praevia:** These include previous caesarean section or uterine surgery, higher parity and increasing maternal age, smoking, cocaine use, multiple pregnancy, previous placenta praevia.

Threatened miscarriage

Obed and Adewole[7] studied the antenatal and labour records of 374 pregnant women who had prior diagnosis of threatened miscarriage, to look for the incidence of placental abruption and placenta praevia. They found that first trimester threatened miscarriage was associated with about two and a half times the risk of placental abruption and placenta praevia compared with that of the general obstetric population. They suggest that women with such a history should be followed closely throughout their pregnancy.

Previous caesarean section

There is evidence from several sources to suggest that women who have had a previous caesarean section are more at risk of developing placenta praevia. Yang et al.,[8] studied a large group of women (n=5 146 742), and found that women who had delivered by caesarean section in their first pregnancy had a 47% risk of placenta praevia and 40% risk of placental abruption in a second singleton pregnancy. Also, the risk of abruption and placenta praevia can increase with the number of previous caesarean sections. Getahun et al.[9] agreed with these findings and added that a short interpregnancy interval, i.e. within one year, is also associated with an increased risk of abruption and placenta praevia.

High parity and older age

Many sources[2,10,11] agree that women who have had three or more previous babies are at higher risk of developing abruption and placenta praevia. In addition, older women of more than 35 years are widely recognised as being more at risk of developing both abruption and placenta praevia.[2,10,11]

Maternal cocaine use

Addis et al.[12] systematically reviewed available data on pregnancy outcome when the mother consumed cocaine. They found that the risk for placental abruption could be statistically related to cocaine use in the pregnant mother.

Smoking

Andres[13] reported that smoking was recognised as having an adverse effect on pregnancy outcome as early as the mid-1950s. He reviewed the published literature written about women who smoked in pregnancy and found that the risk of placental abruption and/or placenta praevia was increased in this group. The risk increased with the number of cigarettes smoked (10 a day or over), and the number of years over which they had smoked (six years or more). Those women who gave up smoking during their pregnancy were shown to be at no greater risk of developing placental abruption than those who didn't smoke.

Hypertensive disorders

It is well documented[14,15] that hypertensive disorders in pregnancy can predispose to placental abruption. Ananth *et al.*[15] reviewed the literature to evaluate the joint influences of smoking and hypertensive disorders (chronic hypertension and pre-eclampsia) on the subsequent development of abruption. They found an increased risk of placental abruption in relation to both smoking and hypertensive disorders during pregnancy. Severe pre-eclampsia and chronic hypertension with superimposed pre-eclampsia have a strong association with placental abruption.[14]

Multiple pregnancy

Another risk factor for both placenta praevia and abruption is multiple pregnancy. Because there is usually a greater surface area of placental tissue with multiple pregnancies, there is more likelihood of it encroaching on the lower segment. Abruption could result after sudden decompression of the uterine cavity, for example after spontaneous rupture of membranes of the first twin, delivery of the first twin, following ECV, or in cases of polyhydramnios.

Domestic violence

Unfortunately, domestic violence is common, occurring in about 1:4 women,

across all social groups, but it is very difficult to quantify. Pregnancy seems to be viewed by violent men as a trigger for further abuse. Violent attacks during pregnancy seem to be focused on the abdomen, breasts and genitals. This is repeatedly shown to be a cause of maternal and perinatal morbidity with an increased risk of placental abruption. Psychological effects on the pregnant woman subjected to domestic violence may lead her to indulge in drug taking, including smoking and alcohol, which, as mentioned, increase the risk of abruption.[16,17]

Uterine rupture

See Chapter 8 for discussion of this condition.

Acute and chronic respiratory diseases in pregnancy

According to Ananth *et al.*,[18] women who require hospitalisation during their pregnancy because of acute and chronic respiratory disease are more likely to experience placental abruption.

Vitamin deficiency

Nilsen *et al.*[19] investigated a possible association of supplemental folic acid and multivitamin use with placental abruption. They studied 280 127 singleton deliveries over a six-year period in Norway and found that those women who had taken vitamin supplements during pregnancy showed a significantly lower risk of developing placental abruption. This could also imply that women from lower socioeconomic groups with poorer nutritional status may also be at higher risk of abruption.

It can be deduced from the lists above that the risks and predisposing factors for abruption and placenta praevia often overlap, but Yang *et al.*[20] found that placental abruption is more likely to be affected by conditions occurring during pregnancy, whereas placenta praevia is more likely to be affected by conditions existing prior to pregnancy.

Placental abruption

Placental abruption occurs in about 1:150 deliveries. It can be defined as the complete or partial separation of a normally implanted placenta occurring after 24 weeks' gestation, prior to delivery, usually accompanied by abdominal pain and uterine bleeding. It is often confirmed after delivery by evidence of retroplacental bleeding or clot.

The perinatal mortality rate with confirmed abruption is high at 30% of those diagnosed. More than half the perinatal losses are due to fetal death before the mother arrives in hospital.[21]

The haemorrhage can be classified (*see* Figure 5.1) as:

- **revealed**: the bleeding usually passes between the membranes and the uterus to escape through the cervix and appear *per vaginum*. This occurs in the majority of cases
- **concealed**: the blood remains trapped between the placenta and the uterus; this is the presentation of 10% of cases
- **mixed**: both of the above occur.

Depending on the degree of separation of the placenta and therefore the condition of the mother and fetus, the severity of the abruption can be described as mild, moderate or severe.

Pathophysiology

Placental separation is triggered by bleeding into the decidua basalis (lining of the uterus) with haematoma formation. The blood clot weighs down and adheres to the maternal surface of the placenta. As the placenta separates, bleeding may track down between the membranes and the uterus and appear externally. This is

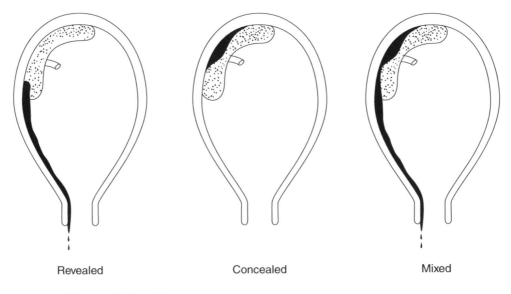

Revealed   Concealed   Mixed

FIGURE 5.1 Placental abruption

a revealed haemorrhage. In a concealed haemorrhage, the bleeding is more centrally located, may be retained behind the placenta and can infiltrate into the myometrium (muscle layer of the uterus), causing pain, uterine tenderness and irritability. If this blood infiltration is significant, it is known as a Couvelaire uterus or uterine apoplexy. A haemorrhage of this severity can lead to fetal and/or maternal death, maternal coagulation defects, renal failure and, rarely, Sheehan's syndrome. A mixed haemorrhage may have some revealed and some concealed bleeding.

Signs and symptoms
Bleeding
As already described, the amount of blood seen when a woman presents with a placental abruption is not associated with the severity of the abruption. Early warning scoring systems may help identify hidden bleeding. The blood may be red if it is fresh loss, but there may be brown blood if it has been retained *in utero* for any length of time.

Shock
The woman's skin may be pale and clammy and her vital signs may suggest hypovolaemic shock. She may also have altered levels of consciousness (*see* Chapter 2 for further discussion).

Abdominal pain
This can be either moderate or severe, intermittent or continuous and of either sudden or gradual onset. Backache may be present if the placenta is posterior and the uterus is generally irritable.

Abdominal examination
In a concealed haemorrhage, there may be an increase in abdominal girth and the uterus may be firm or 'board-like' (Couvelaire) on palpation. The abdomen may be tender to touch.

Evidence of fetal distress
The woman may report a history of reduced or excessive fetal movements. The fetal heart may show signs of distress or be absent.

Anxiety
Any deviation from the norm in the progression of pregnancy can cause anxiety in women.

The abruption may be associated with hypertensive disorders or trauma such as a road traffic accident, attempted external cephalic version or abuse.

Placenta praevia
Placenta praevia is where the placenta is partially or wholly implanted in the lower uterine segment on either the anterior or posterior wall. It occurs in about 0.5% of all pregnancies. The perinatal mortality rate is about 50–60 in every 1000.[21]

Classification divides placenta praevia into four types which can be simplified on clinical grounds to *major* or *minor*[2] (*see* Figure 5.2):

- **Type I (lateral or low-lying)**: the placenta encroaches on the lower uterine segment but does not extend as far as the cervical os.
- **Type II (marginal)**: the edge of the placenta extends to the internal cervical os but does not cover it.
- **Type III (partial)**: the placenta partially covers the internal os.
- **Type IV (complete or central)**: the placenta completely covers the internal os.

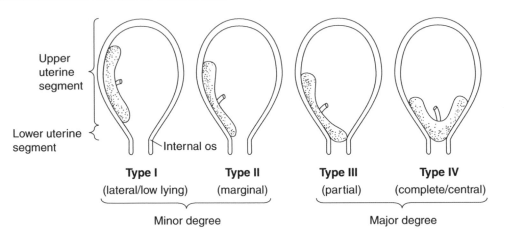

Upper uterine segment

Lower uterine segment

Internal os

Type I
(lateral/low lying)

Type II
(marginal)

Type III
(partial)

Type IV
(complete/central)

Minor degree

Major degree

FIGURE 5.2 Placenta praevia

Approximately half of all placenta praevia are of minor degree (types I and II), and half are major (types III and IV).[11] About 80% of women with placenta praevia bleed before the onset of labour. Generally, those of major degree bleed earlier in the pregnancy and more heavily than those of minor degree.[11] Lam et al.[22] studied the maternal and neonatal outcomes of 159 women with a diagnosed placenta praevia who bled in their pregnancy compared to 93 who did not. They found that the neonatal outcome was worse in those women who had bled, with more respiratory distress, low Apgar scores and admissions to neonatal unit (accounted for mainly by the higher incidence of prematurity). The same women were also more likely to have had antenatal steroids, tocolytic agents and/or emergency caesarean section delivery.

It is commonplace in the UK for pregnant women to have a routine ultrasound scan at 18–20 weeks' gestation. About 5%–6% of all placentae will appear low at this gestation as the lower uterine segment is not yet formed. The NICE guideline for antenatal care[23] recommends that only a woman whose placenta extends over the internal os should be offered another transabdominal scan at 32 weeks. If this scan is then unclear, a transvaginal scan should be offered. She should also be advised what to do if bleeding occurs before this.

Only a minority of the women rescanned will be diagnosed with placenta praevia, and their subsequent management will be decided depending on their individual condition. That means that with placental migration as a result of anatomical changes in the lower segment, 90% of women diagnosed with a low-lying placenta at 20 weeks' gestation will have a normally sited placenta later in pregnancy.[24,25]

Signs and symptoms

With placenta praevia, the placental edge may separate from the uterine wall and cause bleeding which is always visible.

Bleeding

Fresh red blood loss can occur, which is apparently unprovoked. Pain is not a feature because the low-lying placenta allows the blood to escape, thus avoiding the formation of a retroplacental clot.

Bleeding could possibly be initiated by coitus.

Shock

This would correspond to the amount of blood loss. Most healthy pregnant women can tolerate a blood loss of up to 1 litre.[26]

Abdominal palpation

The uterus is usually soft and non-tender. There is often malpresentation and/or unstable lie because the placenta occupies the space in the pelvis where the baby's head usually lies. Breech is particularly common. In any presentation, the presenting part may remain high.

Evidence of fetal distress

The fetal heart is usually normal. Fetal tachycardia may be present and reflect maternal tachycardia. Fetal hypoxia may be present with severe haemorrhage.

Anxiety

Any deviation from the norm in the progression of pregnancy can cause anxiety in women.

Immediate treatment of APH

It is always important to remember that every woman who is experiencing an antepartum haemorrhage is different and should be treated sensitively and individually. A calm attitude and continual explanation of procedures is paramount in order to instil trust and confidence in the woman and her family.

A multidisciplinary standardised approach is essential for optimum care.

Medical aid should be summoned immediately. *See* Box 5.1 for a list of personnel who may be involved. Obviously, the immediate treatment given will depend on the severity of the haemorrhage and therefore the condition of the mother and fetus. Priority should always be given to resuscitating and stabilising the woman before delivering the baby. The midwife should remember that any bleeding can be serious and the condition of the mother and fetus can deteriorate rapidly. If the mother is in pain a narcotic drug may be given.

BOX 5.1 Essential team members for controlling a moderate or severe APH
- Midwife
- Labour ward coordinator
- On-call obstetric team
- Consultant obstetrician
- Blood transfusion service
- Anaesthetist
- Haematologist
- Paediatrician
- Neonatal unit nursing staff
- Porters
- Any other staff to give assistance (such as a scribe) but not get in the way!

Initial observation includes assessment for shock by looking for clammy skin, pallor, air hunger and indications from the woman's vital signs. If the woman with associated hypertension has a placental abruption, her blood pressure may not be abnormally low, thus masking one of the clinical signs of shock.

If the midwife is attending the woman at home, her priority is to transfer her to the nearest consultant-led obstetric unit, ideally with appropriate neonatal facilities. Transfer should be done via the emergency services, by ambulance in accordance with local policies and procedures. An intravenous infusion should be sited to initiate fluid replacement. The mother should be positioned so as to avoid supine hypotension (left lateral tilt), as this could exacerbate her state of shock and further compromise the fetus.

Neither a digital vaginal nor a rectal examination should be performed as this could aggravate the bleeding. A speculum examination may be carried out to exclude cervical or vaginal lesions as a cause for the bleeding, although this procedure may be considered an unnecessary procedure by some obstetricians and midwives. Chilaka *et al.*[27] carried out a study at a UK teaching hospital to determine whether an admission speculum was a necessary routine procedure for all women presenting with antepartum haemorrhage. They found that the complications of pregnancy, timing of delivery and subsequent management were not influenced by the findings from speculum examination. They suggested that this procedure may not be justifiable for all women presenting with antepartum haemorrhage.

Accurate and thorough history taking will give the team information on the amount of blood loss, any associated pain, trauma, recent sexual intercourse or any previous episodes of bleeding. This will help in trying to determine the cause of the bleeding. The woman may have had a recent scan indicating placental location. She may have had previous hospital admissions with bleeding or hypertension.

Palpation will give an indication of the size of the baby and help to determine the cause of haemorrhage according to whether or not the abdomen is tender, soft or 'board-like'. A history of repeated small bleeds during the pregnancy may have resulted in placental insufficiency, which can lead to associated intrauterine growth restriction.

The fetal condition is assessed by initial auscultation, then cardiotocography and a description of the nature of recent fetal movements from the mother.

The blood tests needed are:
- full blood count
- group and cross match/save
- clotting (an additional tube can also be taken and stuck to the wall to observe for signs of clotting while waiting for results – if it doesn't clot within 6–7 minutes there is probably a coagulation problem)
- biochemistry screen in cases of hypertension (*see* Chapter 4 for details of the pre-eclampsia blood tests)
- Kleihauer test (if the mother is rhesus negative).

Intravenous therapy will be administered as necessary to maintain blood pressure and circulating volume.

A scan is necessary in most cases to determine the location of the placenta. Even if this has been done previously in pregnancy, it should be repeated as there have been cases reported where routine pregnancy ultrasound has not been accurate in placental localisation.[11] If the placenta is found to be normally sited, any separation may be seen on ultrasound, although this is not always the case.

See Chapter 10 and Box 10.5 for a description of the preparation necessary if an emergency caesarean section is planned.

Further treatment for APH

Placental abruption

After a **mild** haemorrhage, the condition of the mother and fetus are not normally compromised. The blood loss will probably all be revealed.

If the gestation of the baby is no more than 34 weeks, corticosteroids can be administered to accelerate fetal lung maturity.[28] The woman should be introduced to the neonatal unit staff and a visit to the unit organised. If she is rhesus negative, she should be offered an intramuscular injection of anti-D immunoglobulin with full explanation of its effects. The woman may be allowed home after a period of observation provided there has been no further bleeding, and frequent monitoring indicates that the fetal heart is normal. The placental site will have been determined by ultrasound scan.

If further bleeding occurs and the gestation is 37 weeks or over, labour may be induced. If this coincides with any signs of fetal distress, delivery by caesarean section may be necessary.

A **moderate** haemorrhage is where up to 1 litre of blood has been lost and about one-quarter of the placenta separated. The blood loss may be partially concealed and partially revealed – a mixed haemorrhage. The condition of the mother is compromised with shock, abdominal pain and guarding. Regular observation of these signs, as well as accurate measurements of pulse, oxygen saturations, blood pressure and fluid balance, should be maintained. Analgesia may be required for the mother.

The fetus may have already died or be hypoxic. If it is in good condition or has died, vaginal delivery should be attempted unless there is a contraindication such as transverse lie or malpresentation. The contractions should help to control the bleeding. Enkin *et al.*[29] suggest that inducing labour, using oxytocin if necessary, and continuously monitoring fetal heart rate may result in a 50% reduction of the risk of caesarean section with no significant risk of perinatal mortality.

If the baby is alive but showing signs of distress, caesarean section is the most appropriate mode of delivery once the mother's condition has been stabilised. To treat shock, it is necessary to replace blood loss with appropriate plasma expanders and whole blood so that the baby can be delivered as soon as possible.

With a **severe** haemorrhage, two or more litres of blood may have been lost and more than half of the placenta separated. It is highly likely that the fetus will be dead. The mother will be shocked, in extreme pain and most of the blood will be concealed behind the placenta. The mother may need a central venous pressure line to monitor fluid levels, an indwelling urinary catheter and analgesia. Although the treatment is the same as for a moderate haemorrhage, the mother is more at risk of coagulation defects, renal failure and pituitary failure. Efficient team work and good communication between the labour ward and blood transfusion laboratories are essential.

Placenta praevia

Management decisions for women with placenta praevia are based on clinical and ultrasound findings. Guideline no. 189 in the *International Journal of Gynaecology and Obstetrics*[30] reviewed the use of transvaginal ultrasound (TVS) for the diagnosis of placenta praevia and recommend management based on accurate placental localisation. They suggest that TVS is a safe and more accurate method of scanning than TAS (transabdominal ultrasound) and may reduce hospital stays and unnecessary interventions. The Royal College of Obstetricians and Gynaecologists (RCOG)[24] advocates this method of scanning in their paper on diagnosis and management of placenta praevia. The RCOG[24] suggests that if the placenta encroaches within 2 cm of the internal os, delivery should be by caesarean section. They also specify that the choice of anaesthetic technique must be made by the anaesthetist conducting the procedure.

The first bleed suffered by women with placenta praevia does not normally compromise the mother or fetus and is sometimes referred to as a 'warning bleed'. Severe bleeding usually occurs after the thirty-fourth week of pregnancy and about 50% of women with placenta praevia deliver at less than 35 weeks.[11]

Induction of labour may be appropriate once the fetus has reached an adequate gestation and the placenta has been classified as marginal. However, an artificial rupture of membranes should only be performed in controlled conditions, i.e. in the operating theatre with blood available in case of haemorrhage. The fetal head should be below the placental edge and amniotomy attempted by a senior obstetrician. If any placental tissue can be felt, the procedure should be abandoned and an emergency caesarean section performed.

Expectant or conservative management is appropriate with slight to moderate bleeding. The object is to minimise the problems of prematurity which are possible when a baby is delivered before 37 weeks' gestation. This entails rest in hospital until the bleeding has stopped. The RCOG[24] suggest that women in the third trimester should be hospitalised until delivery if major placenta praevia has been diagnosed. Enkin et al.[29] state that the two randomised trials comparing inpatient and outpatient care for known placenta praevia have not been large enough to permit definite conclusions about safety. Blood must, of course, always be available should the mother bleed again and need an urgent transfusion.

Inpatient treatment includes correction of anaemia in the mother and serial ultrasound scans for fetal well-being. Anti-D and/or steroids should be administered as appropriate (as in placental abruption) and psychological care must be considered. The mother may become institutionalised and miserable with prolonged hospitalisation. She may be separated from other children and need help in organising their care. She may need parentcraft education and a visit to the neonatal unit. A date set for her delivery will give her something positive to focus on.

Possible complications

- **Postpartum haemorrhage:** Following delivery of a woman with APH uncontrollable bleeding may occur despite administration of oxytocics (*see* Chapter 10).
- **Coagulation defects:** The trigger for disseminated intravascular coagulation (DIC) seems to be the entry of tissue thromboplastin or endotoxin into the circulation, inducing thrombin activation. A consumption coagulopathy occurs where fibrinogen, coagulation factors and circulating platelets are depleted. The result is haemostatic failure with microvascular bleeding and an

increased blood loss. DIC can arise from APH and haemorrhagic shock (*see* Chapter 10 and Box 10.9 for further discussion of the diagnosis and management of DIC).

- **Anaemia:** A result of excessive blood loss, anaemia may require correction by blood transfusion or oral iron therapy. The RCOG[24] recommends that possible blood transfusion requirements are discussed with all women with placenta praevia and their partners prior to delivery to ensure that any objections or queries are dealt with effectively. Bonner[21] suggests that every unit should establish specific protocols for the management of women who refuse blood.
- **Infection:** Infection may be acquired through low resistance caused by shock, anaemia or through increased interventions.
- **Renal failure:** Renal failure may occur as a result of severe shock.
- **Hysterectomy:** This can result from uncontrollable haemorrhage, particularly as a result of Couvelaire uterus or coagulation defects.
- **Sheehan's syndrome:** Anterior pituitary necrosis or Sheehan's syndrome is a rare complication of prolonged shock. It can result in failure of lactation, amenorrhoea, hypothyroidism and adrenocortical insufficiency following the pregnancy.
- **Fetal hypoxia:** Fetal hypoxia may occur as a result of premature placental separation.
- **Premature delivery and resulting sequelae:** Any delivery occurring between 24 and 37 weeks' gestation as a result of placental abruption or placenta praevia will require varying

degrees of input from the neonatal unit. Long-term follow-up may ensue and need input from the community and social services.
- **Fetal death:** Death of the fetus is rare but more common in abruption.[1]

Adverse psychological effects

Adverse psychological effects, such as post-natal depression or post-traumatic stress disorder (*see* Chapter 13 for additional discussion of these issues) could occur as a result of prolonged periods of hospitalisation, a traumatic delivery or negative fetal outcome. Midwives can help by generally debriefing and providing support if the baby is in the neonatal unit. It may be necessary to refer the mother for bereavement counselling and she may wish to receive advice on the risks for subsequent pregnancies (for example, the recurrence rate for placenta praevia is 4%–8%).

Morbidly adherent placenta (placenta accrete, increta and percreta)

Because of the rise in caesarean section rates, the incidence of placenta accreta is rising.[31] See further discussion in the section on 'Morbidly adherent placenta' in Chapter 10.

Checklist: what to do when an APH occurs

In hospital some of the actions below will be done simultaneously because many personnel may be involved. Antepartum haemorrhage requires immediate action.
- Assess clinical situation and perform cardiopulmonary resuscitation if necessary.

- Arrange transfer to hospital by ambulance if at home.
- Ensure appropriate personnel assembled.
- Establish venous access and administer fluids.
- Continuous assessment of maternal and fetal condition.
- Replace blood loss as necessary.
- Maintain fluid balance records.
- Collect blood samples.
- Give analgesia as necessary.
- Deliver baby (if necessary) after mother stabilised.
- Documentation: time, action, reaction.
- Continual explanation and calm attitude.
- Consideration of long-term psychological complications (*see* Chapter 13).

References

1 Siddiqui F, Kean L. (2009) Intrauterine fetal death. *Obstet Gynaecol Reprod Med.* **19**(1): 1–6.

2 Sinha P, Kuruba N. (2008) Antepartum haemorrhage: an update. *J Obstet Gynaecol.* **28**(4): 377–81.

3 Hall J. (2005) Midwifery basics: complications in pregnancy (1) Antepartum haemorrhage. *Pract Midwife.* **8**(9): 29–32.

4 Hamilton-Fairley D. (2009) '*Diseases of pregnancy*' in Obstetrics and Gynaecology. 3rd ed. London: Wiley-Blackwell.

5 McCormack RA, *et al.* (2008) Antepartum bleeding of unknown origin in the second half of pregnancy and pregnancy outcomes. *BJOG.* **115**(11): 1451–7.

6 Lewis G, editor. (2007) *CEMACH Saving mothers lives: reviewing maternal deaths to make motherhood safer 2003–2005. The seventh report on the confidential enquiries into maternal deaths in the United Kingdom.* London: RCOG Press.

7 Obed J, Adewole I. (1996) Antepartum haemorrhage: the influence of first trimester uterine bleeding. *West Afr J Med.* **15**(1): 61–3.

8 Yang Q, Wen SW, *et al.* (2007) Association of caesarean delivery for first birth with placenta previa and placental abruption in second pregnancy. *BJOG.* **114**: 609–13.

9 Getahun D, *et al.* (2006) Previous caesarean delivery and risks of placenta previa and placental abruption. *Obstet Gynecol.* **107**(4): 771–8.

10 Abu-Heija AT, El-Jallad F, Ziadeh S. (1999) Placenta praevia: effect of age, gravidity, parity and previous caesarean section. *Gynecol Obstet Invest.* **47**(1): 6–8.

11 Baskett TF. (2004) *Antepartum Haemorrhage in Essential Management of Obstetric Emergencies.* Bristol: Clinical Press Ltd.

12 Addis A, Moretti ME, *et al.* (2001) Fetal effects of cocaine: an updated meta-analysis. *Reprod Toxicol.* **15**(4): 341–69.

13 Andres RL. (1996) The association of cigarette smoking with placenta praevia and abruptio placentae. *Semin Perinatol.* **20**(2): 154–9.

14 Powrie R, Rosene-Montella K. (2008) Pre-eclampsia. In: Rosene-Montella K, Keely E, Barbour L, Lee R. *Medical Care of the Pregnant Patient.* Philadelphia: ACP Press.

15 Ananth CV, Smulian JC, Vintzileos AM. (1999) Incidence of placental abruption in relation to cigarette smoking and hypertensive disorders during pregnancy: a metaanalysis of observational studies. *J Obstet Gynaecol.* **4**: 662–8.

16 Hunt S, Martin AM. (2001) *Pregnant Women, Violent Men: what midwives need to know.* Oxford: Books for Midwives Press.

17 Rachana C. Suraiya K, *et al.* (2002) Prevalence and complications of physical violence during pregnancy. *Eur J Obstet Gynecol Reprod Biol.* **103**(1): 26–9.

18 Ananth CV, *et al.* (2006) Acute and chronic respiratory diseases in pregnancy: associations with placental abruption. *Am J Obstet Gynecol.* **195**(4): 1180–4.

19 Nilsen RM, Vollset SE, *et al.* (2008) Folic acid and multivitamin supplement use and risk of placental abruption: a population-based registry study. *Am J Epidemiol.* **167**(7): 867–74.

20 Yang Q, Wen SW, *et al.* (2009) Comparison of maternal risk factors between placental abruption and placental praevia. *Am J Perinatol.* **26**(4): 279–86.

21 Bonner J. (2000) Massive obstetric haemorrhage. In: Arulkumaran S, editor. *Emergencies in Obstetrics and Gynaecology.* London: Baillière Tindall.

22 Lam CM, Wong SF, Chow KM, *et al.* (2000) Women with placenta praevia and antepartum haemorrhage have a worse outcome than those who do not bleed before delivery. *J Obstet Gynaecol.* **20**(1): 27–31.

23 National Institute for Health and Clinical Excellence (NICE). (2008) *Clinical Guideline 62: antenatal care: routine care for healthy pregnant women.* London: NICE Publications.

24 Paterson-Brown S. (2005) *Placenta Praevia and Placenta Praevia Accreta: diagnosis and management Guideline 27.* London: RCOG Press.

25 Farine D, Keenan-Lindsay L, Morin V, *et al.* (2007) Diagnosis and management of placenta praevia. *Int J Gynecol Obstet.* **103**(1): 89–94.

26 Steele D. (2007) Haemorrhagic disorders and the critically ill woman. In: Billington M, Stevenson M, editors. *Critical Care in Childbirth for Midwives.* Oxford: Blackwell Publishing.

27 Chilaka VN, Konje JC, Clarke S, *et al.* (2000) Practice observed: is speculum examination on admission a necessary procedure in the management of all cases of antepartum haemorrhage? *J Obstet Gynaecol.* **20**(4): 396–8.

28 Crowley P. (2001) Prophylactic steroids for preterm birth. *Cochrane Database Syst Rev.* **2**: CD000065.

29 Enkin M, Keirse M, Neilson JP, *et al.* editors. (2000) *A Guide to Effective Care in Pregnancy and Childbirth.* 3rd ed. Oxford: Oxford University Press.

30 International Journal of Gynaecology and Obstetrics. (2007) Diagnosis and management of placenta praevia: guideline no. 189. *Int J Gynaecol Obstet.* **103**(1): 89–94.

31 Oelese Y, Smulian JC. (2006) Placenta previa, placenta accreta and vasa previa. *Obstet Gynecol.* **107**(4) 927–41.

CHAPTER 6

Malpresentations and malpositions

Judith Robbins

The definition of *malpresentation* refers to the fetus presenting other than by the vertex. This includes, most commonly, breech and, more rarely, face, brow, compound and shoulder. In addition there are the non-longitudinal presentations, namely transverse or oblique lies.

The term *malposition* describes the fetus presenting by the vertex whereby the occiput (the denominator) is facing the posterior of the pelvis.

The midwife will frequently identify and manage the care of women with malpositions and, less frequently, diagnose and refer women with malpresentations. It is vital that the midwife is aware that these situations frequently result in prolonged or obstructed labour and emergency delivery.

Breech presentation

Breech is a malpresentation where there is longitudinal lie of the fetus with the buttocks in the lower pole of the uterus. The denominator is the sacrum and the presenting diameter is bitrochanteric (10 cm). At 28 weeks' gestation the

incidence of breech is approximately 20%. Spontaneous version reduces this percentage to approximately 3%–4% at term.[1]

Classification
There are three types of breech presentation.
- **Frank or extended breech:** this occurs most frequently (70%) in primiparous women who have firm abdominal muscles. The extended breech presents with flexion at the hips and extension at the knees so that the feet are lying near the fetal head. This results in a well-fitting presenting part (*see* Figure 6.1a).
- **Complete (flexed) breech:** this results in a poor-fitting presenting part, presenting with flexion at the hips and the knees with feet beside the buttocks. The risks are early rupture of the membranes and cord prolapse (*see* Figure 6.1b).
- **Footling breech:** the rarest type of breech, this has one or both feet or knees presenting. There is extension at the hip(s) and knee(s). There is

a high risk of cord prolapse as the presenting part is so ill-fitting (*see* Figure 6.1c).

Predisposing factors and underlying pathophysiology

In many cases there is no obvious cause for a malpresentation or malposition. Factors that may increase the incidence of breech include prematurity or intrauterine growth restriction. Before 34 weeks' gestation the fetus has more room to manoeuvre *in utero*. Both factors can result in the breech birth of a low birth weight baby, which is in itself an indicator for poor perinatal outcome.[2]

Multiple pregnancy carries an increased risk of breech because the space for one or more fetuses to turn is reduced and multiple pregnancy is, in itself, a risk for preterm labour.

Major fetal abnormalities such as hydrocephaly also predispose to breech presentation. In such cases the fetal head is thought to be better accommodated in the fundus of the uterus. The fetus also has more room to move when the uterus is distended as in the case of polyhydramnios, which also carries the increased risk of cord prolapse. Conversely, oligohydramnios may predispose to breech where, because of the small amount of fluid, fetal movement is restricted and the fetus is 'trapped' in the presentation assumed in the second trimester.[3,4]

Maternal intake of substances that may cause the fetus to reduce its movements (for example anticonvulsive medication or alcohol) can also predispose to breech presentation.[5]

Maternal factors thought to influence the incidence of breech presentation include any space-occupying uterine abnormalities. Examples include the presence of a septum or partial septum (bicornuate uterus), or in rare cases the presence of uterine neoplasms such as leiomyomata. Similarly, the presence of fibroids or pelvic tumours and placental implantation in the lower uterine segment (placenta praevia) is thought to contribute to the aetiology of breech presentation.[5] All these anomalies reduce uterine space for fetal movement and/or prevent the fetal head entering the pelvis.[6]

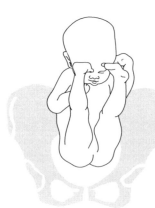
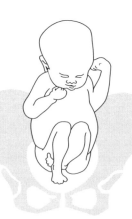
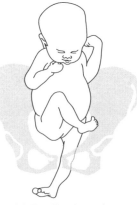

(a) Frank breech   (b) Complete breech   (c) Footling breech

FIGURE 6.1a, b, c Classification of breech presentations

Grand multiparity may lead to an increased rate of breech presentation as lax abdominal muscles give the fetus more room to move. It is thought that women with a history of caesarean delivery may also predispose to breech presentation.[7]

Research carried out in the USA cites maternal diabetes, older maternal age, smoking during pregnancy, primiparity and late or no prenatal care as all carrying an increased risk of breech presentation.[8] The authors discuss the possibility of several different factors and biological mechanisms interacting to increase the rate of breech.

Consideration should also be given to the fact that some women deliver all their babies as breeches, suggesting that their pelvic shape is better suited to a breech. Although pelvic classification is controversial, obstetric texts frequently refer to an increased risk of breech with some pelvic shapes. Examples include the platypelloid (anteroposteriorly flat) and android (heart-shaped); both these physiques make cephalic pelvic entry more difficult than in pelves with more favourable configurations.

Diagnosis and reducing the incidence of breech presentation

Breech presentation carries higher rates of perinatal mortality and morbidity than cephalic presentation.[9] A common complication of a breech presentation is a prolapsed cord. The incidence of prolapsed cord is increased when the fetus is small (often premature or growth restricted) or the presenting breech is ill-fitting, but differs with each type of breech. With a frank breech the incidence is approximately 0.5%, which is similar to the rate found in cephalic presentations. The rate obviously increases for complete breech presentations and for footling/knee presentations (see Chapter 7 for further information on cord prolapse).

Abdominal examination

Breech presentation is commonly diagnosed by abdominal palpation, although this is not always easy and may often need to be confirmed by ultrasound. A history of breech presentations or the presence of any of the aforementioned predisposing factors can sometimes alert the midwife to the possibility of a breech. On inspection there may be little to see; the lie is longitudinal and on palpation the uterine size may palpate larger than expected for dates. This is due to the fact that the breech may not have entered the pelvis. Using a Pawlik's grip, the head is located in the fundus and felt as a round hard mass, which may move independently of the back by ballotting it with one or both hands. However, in a frank breech, if the feet are 'splinting' the head, the diagnosis may not be easily made.

Both poles of the fetus may be grasped simultaneously to aid diagnosis and if the entire breech is moveable above the pelvis it may be assumed that the fetal pelvis has not passed through the maternal pelvic inlet. Typically, the fetal back is felt on one side of the abdomen and the fetal small parts on the other. Mothers with breech presentation often complain of discomfort under the ribs and heartburn caused by the proximity of the fetal head.

On auscultation fetal heart sounds are often heard best at or above the umbilicus and laterally on the side of the fetal back.

Posture

Much has been written regarding the use in pregnancy of the knee–chest all-fours position as a means of encouraging spontaneous version from breech to cephalic presentation.[10] Evidence from a Cochrane review describes how uncontrolled trials encourage women to adopt the knee–chest position for varying time periods in late pregnancy. The review concludes that these studies show no significant benefit for breech version.[11] Smith *et al.*[10] reported no benefits in the use of postural management and saw no reason to recommend it. However, midwifery care emphasizes psychological as well as physical benefits and so where no adverse consequences have been proved, the active involvement of the mother may well be beneficial to her. This must be balanced against the mother possibly feeling disappointed and guilty if the baby does not turn, as identified in Kariminia's research[12] with occipitoposterior (OP) positions.

Complementary therapies

There is some evidence that an acupuncture technique using moxibustion can be used to turn breech presentations and women may choose to access these services.[13,14]

External cephalic version (ECV)

It has been the RCOG[9] audit standard for some time to offer ECV to women with an uncomplicated breech presentation at term.[15] This procedure is the manipulative transabdominal conversion of the breech to cephalic presentation and is successful for about 50% of all women. ECV is generally safe, although it is recommended that the procedure should always be undertaken in a place where a baby can be delivered by emergency caesarean section if necessary. Transient fetal heart rate anomalies post procedure may occur in approximately 1:300 cases;

and placental abruption is rare occurring in 1:1000 cases.[9] Overall, there is a significant reduction in the risk of caesarean section in women undergoing this procedure without any increased risk to the fetus. The procedure should not be commenced if there has been recent vaginal bleeding, rupture of membranes, multiple pregnancy or the woman is known to have a bicornuate uterus.[16]

Prior to the obstetrician performing an ECV, the woman must be fully informed of the risks and understand the procedure itself and her consent documented. A normal fetal heart rate must be recorded on the CTG. An ultrasound examination is performed to determine fetal position, position of the legs, head flexion and liquor volume. A tocolytic is then administered; for example terbutaline.[9] The procedure involves the woman lying flat with a wedge tilt or on her side with the fetal back upwards. Using the palmer surfaces of both hands, the fetal breech is disengaged from the pelvis by the obstetrician. Once disengaged, the breech is gently pulled upward and laterally to allow fetal flexion and the fetus 'follows its nose'. The whole procedure should be gentle and unrushed.

The midwife should be constantly aware of any discomfort, as the procedure can be painful,[16] and Entonox® may be used. The fetal heart should be auscultated between each attempt (a maximum of three attempts). The midwife must repeat the CTG post procedure and if the woman is rhesus negative, blood for Kleihauer should be taken and anti-D administered. If the ECV has been successful, signs of spontaneous labour should be discussed, together with precautionary awareness of vaginal bleeding or reduced fetal movements. If unsuccessful, plans should be made by the obstetrician for mode of delivery or a possible repeat attempt at a later date.

Labour

It is not uncommon for a woman who has accessed regular antenatal care to arrive in labour with an unknown breech presentation, and this may be first diagnosed by the admitting midwife. Approximately 10% of breech presentations at term will be undetected.[5] All midwives should be alert to the possibility of earlier palpations and vaginal examinations being incorrect, and undertake each assessment without preconceived ideas.

Vaginal examination (VE)

An abdominal palpation prior to the VE will present as described above. On vaginal examination, the smooth head with its landmarks is absent. The presenting part is often high, is soft and irregular, and sometimes the anal orifice can be felt. If landmarks can be felt, in a breech they will be in a line (e.g. fetal ischial tuberosities and the anus), although in a very compressed breech, the cleft between buttocks may be mistaken for the sagittal suture. After rupture of the membranes, fresh meconium can often be noted, especially on the examining finger following identification of the anus, and this is diagnostic. The midwife may also feel a foot or, in rare circumstances, a knee. However, vaginal diagnosis of breech, particularly in early labour, is sometimes difficult and mistakes can be made.

Mechanism of labour: left sacro-anterior (LSA)

- Longitudinal lie.
- Attitude of flexion.
- Breech presentation.
- Position LSA.

- Denominator is the sacrum.
- The presenting part is the anterior left buttock.
- Engagement takes place when the bitrochanteric diameter has passed through the inlet of the pelvis.
- Descent takes place with increasing compaction. Since the breech is a less efficient dilator than the head, descent is usually slow (a sign that should alert the midwife when presentation is unsure).
- Flexion: lateral flexion takes place at the waist. The anterior hip becomes the leading part.
- Internal rotation of the buttocks: the anterior buttock reaches the resistance of the pelvic floor and rotates forward to lie underneath the symphysis pubis.
- Increased lateral flexion occurs as the anterior buttock impinges under the symphysis pubis. With further descent the buttocks are born and rise up the perineum.
- Following expulsion of the legs the buttocks then fall towards the maternal anus.
- The anterior buttock restitutes to the right.
- The shoulders enter the pelvis in the left oblique. The anterior shoulder rotates forward toward the symphysis pubis and is born. The posterior shoulder follows.
- As the shoulders are at the outlet the head enters the pelvis. It enters with the sagittal suture in the transverse diameter of the brim. The occiput meets the pelvic floor and rotates forward so that the sagittal suture is in the anteroposterior diameter.
- The sacrum rotates towards the pubis so the back is anterior.

- As the nape of the neck pivots under the symphysis, the chin, mouth, nose, forehead and occiput are born by flexion.

Breech delivery

The first action of a midwife when confronted by an unexpected breech delivery must be to call for help. This would be either for medical assistance within a hospital setting or for emergency services in the community. Professional backup is imperative in both situations.

Position for delivery should be discussed with the woman. The most common position is semi-recumbent with space at the end of the bed to allow the baby to hang.[9] Upright positions are controversial,[5] but some midwives will suggest a position on hands and knees.[17]

Full dilatation of the cervix must be confirmed before encouraging the woman to push. This will prevent the head from becoming trapped within a partially dilated cervix. If this occurs, a retractor or finger can be used to push aside the cervix to clear an airway in the vagina for the baby's nose or mouth. Delivery must then be expedited.

The age-old principle underpinning breech delivery is still valid: **hands off the breech**. Any handling of the baby is liable to stimulate premature respiration, and therefore touching should only be done if necessary.

The baby's legs should deliver spontaneously, but if necessary they can be assisted by placing two fingers along the length of one thigh with the fingertips in the popliteal fossa. Each leg is then flexed across the body and down.

Once the baby has birthed to the umbilicus and the legs have been delivered, a loop of cord may be brought down to reduce cord tension, although this is rarely necessary. Unnecessary handling of the cord should of course be strictly avoided. The baby's body should be loosely draped in a warm towel to prevent heat loss, as cold could also stimulate respiration.

If necessary the midwife can assess the position of the baby's arms by placing her fingers on the baby's chest. If she can feel elbows, the arms are flexed and should deliver with the next contraction. However, if the arms are extended the Løvset manoeuvre is necessary to continue the delivery. If traction has been used during the delivery, it is likely the arms will be extended. This is one reason to avoid traction and indeed any unnecessary handling during a breech delivery.

Løvset manoeuvre

Holding the baby at the hip bones with the thumbs over the sacrum, downward traction must be applied in combination with rotation. Care must be taken to always keep the fetal back towards the mother's front (i.e. the fetal back must be uppermost if the woman is in a semi-recumbent position). The baby is then rotated 180 degrees so as to splint the posterior arm across the baby's face and change it to an anterior position.

If the arm does not then deliver spontaneously, the midwife should draw it gently down over the chest by flexing the elbow with her finger. The baby is then rotated back in the opposite direction and the second arm is delivered (*see* Figure 6.2).

Delivery of the head

The head must be allowed to move through the pelvis in a transverse position until it rotates spontaneously to bring the

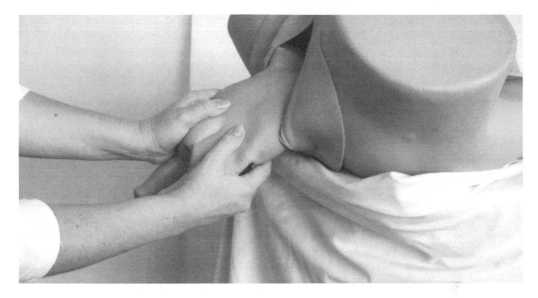

FIGURE 6.2 Løvset manoeuvre for delivery of extended arms

occiput under the symphysis pubis with the back anterior. The head can then be delivered by one of two manoeuvres (or by forceps).

- **Burns Marshall manoeuvre:**
  with the baby's back towards the mother's front (i.e. the baby's back is uppermost if the woman is semi-recumbent), the baby can be allowed to hang without support. This brings the head down onto the perineum. After a brief time, the hairline will appear and the sub-occipital region can be felt. The midwife will then grasp the baby's ankles and while maintaining traction, pivot the sub-occipital region through an arc of 180 degrees until the mouth and nose are free at the vulva. The perineum is guarded with the midwife's other hand to prevent sudden escape of the head, and the mother is then encouraged to breathe out the remainder of the head, thus preventing sudden changes in

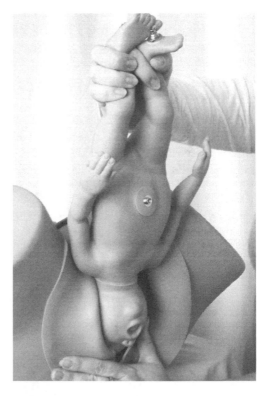

FIGURE 6.3 Burns Marshall method of delivering the after-coming head of a breech presentation

pressure. As the face is born, suction may be applied to clear the airway. Care must also be taken not to overstretch or compress the baby's spine (*see* Figure 6.3).

- **Mauriceau-Smellie-Veit manoeuvre:** for a non-flexed head. The baby's body is laid along the midwife's arm with the palm held upwards supporting the chest. The index and ring fingers of that hand are placed on the malar bones of the baby's face and the middle finger on the baby's chin. This draws the jaw downwards and increases flexion. The midwife should then place her other hand across the baby's shoulders with her middle fingers on the occiput to increase flexion. The head is drawn out until the sub-occipital region appears and the head is pivoted around the symphysis pubis (*see* Figure 6.4). This manoeuvre is also used when the fetal head is extended and descent is delayed. The risk of overstretching or compression of the fetal spine during the Burns Marshall manoeuvre may be avoided. As before, with the Burns Marshall manoeuvre when the face is born, suction may be applied to clear the airway.

- **Emergency breech extraction:** this is rarely undertaken, and only as an emergency procedure to achieve immediate delivery of the baby when there is severe fetal distress or to deliver a second twin in a transverse or oblique lie after internal podalic version. This is therefore a procedure usually undertaken by an obstetrician. A hand must be placed into the uterus and if possible both feet grasped. The legs must be pulled down and the head pressed upwards with the outside hand. Traction

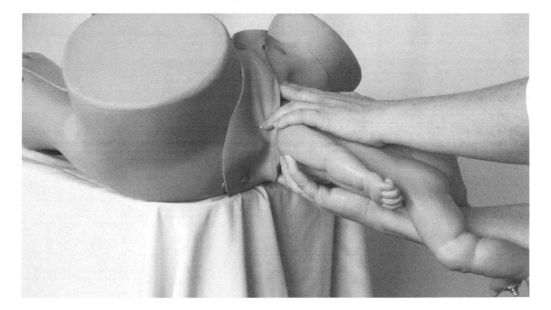

FIGURE 6.4 Mauriceau-Smellie-Veit manoeuvre for delivering the after-coming head of a breech presentation

must be maintained on the delivered legs until the breech is fixed (*see* Figure 6.5). Traction takes the place of contractions and the breech can then be delivered by the methods set out above.[5] As the arms will be extended following traction, Løvset's manoeuvre will be necessary to deliver the arms.

The breech delivery at home

There is a paucity of recent literature outlining risk and outcomes for planned breech births taking place at home. However, choice of venue is something all mothers should have, having first been informed and guided by up-to-date and sound evidence. In addition, choice must include different birth options and settings within the hospital environment.[18–20]

However, experience of breech birth at home is fast becoming a rarity, as rising caesarean section rates reduce opportunities for midwives and doctors to gain skills in the delivery of vaginal breeches.[21–23] This trend de-skills midwives as they lose not only the opportunity for hands-on experience, but also opportunities to observe vaginal breech delivery. However, all midwives must maintain a good knowledge of breech delivery procedures as the chance of an undiagnosed and therefore unexpected breech presentation in second stage does exist.

Besides having the necessary skills to enable a safe delivery, priorities for the midwife are to obtain help, maintain a calm environment and prepare for potential maternal PPH or neonatal resuscitation. The environment must be kept warm to prevent neonatal hypothermia and ensuing hypoglycaemia. Early feeding is highly desirable.

The breech delivery in hospital

The same priorities as above apply. However, preparing for a breech delivery in hospital is now usually associated with preparation for surgery.

Although it is not within the scope of this chapter to discuss the evidence on choice of mode of breech delivery,

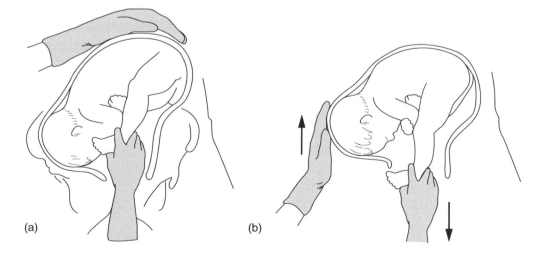

(a) (b)

FIGURE 6.5a, b Breech extraction presentations

it is important to note current trends based on research. Literature examining outcomes following vaginal versus caesarean breech delivery is abundant, but often contradictory. A very influential international randomised controlled trial (the Hannah *et al.* trial)[24] attested to the significantly lower rates of perinatal mortality, neonatal mortality and serious neonatal morbidity when planned caesarean section is carried out as opposed to vaginal birth. No differences were noted in terms of serious maternal morbidity and the primary recommendation is for breech presentations to be delivered by caesarean section. This trial is not beyond criticism[25] and many questions regarding the protocol have been asked, for example

about the positions that the women in the vaginal mode group were encouraged to adopt.[26] However, the Hannah *et al.* trial will further increase the rate of caesarean sections carried out for breech presentations, inevitably contributing to a de-skilling of birth attendants involved in vaginal breech delivery. These controversies emphasise that it is imperative for midwives to keep themselves well informed with up-to-date information. The midwife must be able to competently deliver a breech, whether it is undiagnosed until the sight of the buttocks, or for a woman who chooses a vaginal breech birth. *See* Box 6.1 for a checklist of possible actions when undertaking a vaginal breech delivery.

BOX 6.1 Vaginal breech delivery checklist

- Abdominal palpation.
- Vaginal examination to assess cervical full dilatation.
- Ensure woman is positioned appropriately.
- Regular auscultation.
- 'Hands off the breech.'
- Possible assistance in delivery of extended legs.
- Release loop of cord if necessary, otherwise avoid handling.
- Check for position of arms.
- Drape the baby in a towel to keep it warm.
- Keep the baby's back to the mother's front (i.e. back uppermost if woman is in semi-recumbent position).

- Løvset manoeuvre for arm/shoulder delivery if necessary.
- Allow descent of the head through pelvis (avoidance of traction will ensure the head remains flexed) and spontaneous rotation to occipitoanterior (OA).
- Slow delivery of the head using Burns Marshall or Mauriceau-Smellie-Veit manoeuvre.
- Possible suction and neonatal resuscitation.
- Appropriate third stage management.
- Maintain the baby's temperature.
- Early feeding.
- Paediatric assessment.

Possible complications of vaginal breech delivery

Baby

- Fractures of the humerus, clavicle or femur
- Dislocation of the hip or shoulder
- Erb's palsy
- Internal organ damage by rough or faulty handling (e.g. kidneys, liver, spleen)
- Dislocation of the neck
- Spinal cord damage or spinal fracture
- Intracranial haemorrhage
- Soft-tissue damage
- Hypoxia, birth asphyxia; this may be due to cord compression, cord prolapse or premature placental separation
- Cold injury and hypoglycaemia
- Long-term neurological damage
- Congenital dislocation of the hip, especially with extended breech; this is usually a complication of the presentation, not the birth process.

Mother

- Urethral trauma
- Vaginal or perineal trauma
- PPH.

Conclusion

Breech presentation carries increased risks to mother and baby. Midwives must not only develop and maintain their skills for emergency delivery but also focus on the psychological impact of such a birth. Evidence-informed theory underpins practice and compassionate empathy underpins the art of midwifery. In combination, both allow midwives to provide the unique care that only they can give.

Transverse or oblique lie

Transverse and oblique lie are usually part of an unstable lie, when the fetus moves between longitudinal, transverse and oblique after 37 weeks.[27] The baby may lie directly in the transverse or in the oblique with head or breech in the iliac fossa (*see* Figure 6.6).

Transverse lie occurs when the long axes of mother and fetus are at right angles to one another. The presenting part is most frequently the shoulder. Transverse lie is best dealt with antenatally where appropriate care can be planned to avoid the emergency situation.

Causes

Maternal causes include lax uterine muscles as seen in multiparity and uterine anomalies such as a bicornuate or sub-septate uterus. Low-lying fibroids, placenta praevia and a contracted pelvis also increase the risk.

Fetal causes include prematurity and polyhydramnios (where the fetus has more room to change position), fetal macrosomia and fetal abnormality. Transverse lie is common for the second baby in a twin pregnancy.

Signs and symptoms
Abdominal palpation

Diagnosis is usually made antenatally. On inspection the uterus appears broad and on palpation no poles, for example the head or breech, are felt in the pelvis or fundus. The woman may experience discomfort when the lower segment is touched. In labour, if the shoulder becomes wedged in the pelvis, labour is obstructed and the uterine contractions may become tonic so no relaxation of the uterus can be felt. If operative delivery is not expedited uterine rupture, death of

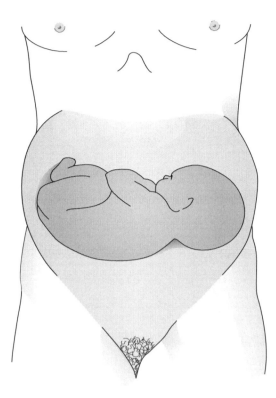

(a) Transverse lie

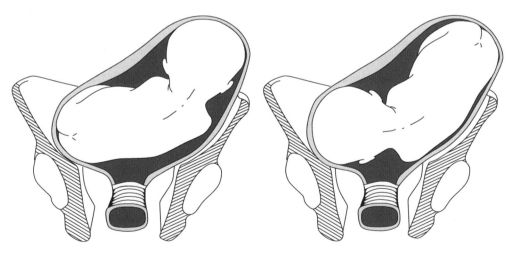

Breech in iliac fossa   Head in iliac fossa

(b) Oblique lie

FIGURE 6.6a, b Transverse and oblique lie

the fetus and/or possible maternal death will ensue.

Vaginal examination

Often little is felt on examination as the presenting part is high. If the midwife discovers a shoulder, she may feel a soft irregular mass or even the ribs. It is possible the arm may have prolapsed through the cervix, and the midwife will feel this – it can be distinguished from a prolapsed leg, by identifying the heel of the foot, or the flexibility of the thumb of the hand. With a high presenting part the risk of cord prolapse is high. There is no mechanism for vaginal delivery of shoulder presentation.

Risks

Maternal risks include prolonged/obstructed labour, fistula formation, infection from prolonged ruptured membranes, uterine rupture and psychological trauma.

Fetal/infant risks include bony and/or soft-tissue injury, hypoxia and/or intrauterine death.

Emergency management

- Call for medical assistance.
- Urgently transfer to hospital if at home.
- If the membranes rupture, check for cord prolapse (*see* Chapter 7).
- Prepare for delivery by caesarean section (and in some cases a classical incision may be necessary)[27]. In cases where facilities for caesarean do not exist or with a second twin delivery, internal podalic version may be attempted with the baby delivered as a footling breech. However, this is dangerous with high rates of neonatal mortality and morbidity.[27]

Occipitoposterior position
Definition and incidence

Occipitoposterior positioning occurs when the fetal occiput is malpositioned in the posterior of the pelvis. More often than not, OP positions turn spontaneously. However, about 20%–35% of those who begin labour in an OP position do not rotate, and approximately 1%–5% deliver vaginally as OP.[27] As outcomes can differ with this position, labour is frequently prolonged and failure to progress may occur.

Predisposing factors and underlying pathophysiology

In most cases the aetiology of this malposition is unknown. However, women with a previous history of OP are more likely to suffer a repeat.[28] It has also been suggested that a contracted pelvis predisposes to OP with the occiput occupying the more spacious hindpelvis. A study by Gardberg *et al.*[29] demonstrated that 68% of persistent OP positions developed through a malrotation during labour from an initially anterior position. There has also been much discussion about the role of maternal positioning and sedentary lifestyles in determining the position of the fetus.[30]

Reducing the incidence of occipitoposterior

Randomised controlled trials to assess the impact of midwifery interventions on OP position are inconclusive. However, discussions of potential methods to help women are readily available.[30] One suggestion is that the woman should assume a position on all fours with raised buttocks prior to and during labour. This position tilts the pelvis forward, maximising the angle between the spine and pelvis, and therefore the space available to enable the baby's head to engage more easily.[31,32]

During labour, the deflexed head in an OP position is often poorly applied to the cervix. Stimulation of oxytocin is reduced and labour is often slow. With modern management this type of labour is frequently augmented via amniotomy and Syntocinon. El Halta[33] suggests that this is the worst thing that can be done as ruptured membranes encourage descent, limiting the opportunity for rotation and predisposing to deep transverse arrest. With membranes intact, the mother can assume a position on all fours with the buttocks raised, which may encourage the head to rotate to an anterior position, with the amniotic fluid providing a cushion for the head.[34] Internal manual rotation to an anterior position has been suggested by Reichman.[35] This technique involves placing fingers on the sagittal suture line, applying pressure to disengage the head and then turning the fingers to rotate the baby. This is not recommended for the inexperienced midwife, but may be more appropriate when recourse to medical assistance is not available and delivery needs to be expedited.

Signs and symptoms
Abdominal palpation

Occipitoposterior position should be considered if engagement has not occurred at term in the primiparous woman. This is because the OP position makes it more difficult for the fetus to negotiate the pelvis.

The fetal back may be difficult to find or is found to be in a lateral position. The fetal head is posterior-lateral and not engaged. A dip is often noted at the mother's umbilicus, marking the space between the baby's arms and legs. The fetal heartbeat is heard laterally or at the umbilicus.

Labour and vaginal examination

Labour may be slow or prolonged and the mother may complain of excessive back pain. Early rupture of the membranes is common, especially if the presenting part is ill-fitting. OP is confirmed if the midwife locates the anterior fontanelle in the anterior during a vaginal examination. However, vaginal examination can be complicated by the presence of caput succedaneum and moulding.

Possible outcomes of labour
Long internal rotation

If engagement occurs in the right oblique diameter of the brim, descent occurs in the right oblique diameter as a right occipitoposterior position. Descent continues to the pelvic floor and progress depends on flexion of the head. If flexion increases and the occiput meets the resistance of the pelvic floor, it will rotate anteriorly through 135 degrees (three-eighths of a circle) to a direct occipitoanterior position and then birth occurs as in the usual OA position.

Short internal rotation

If engagement occurs in the right oblique diameter of the brim, descent occurs in the right oblique diameter as a right occipitoposterior position. Descent continues to the pelvic floor and progress again depends on flexion of the head. If the fetal head is deflexed and remains that way, the sinciput reaches the resistance of the pelvic floor and rotates forward. The occiput settles into the hollow of the sacrum and the fetal chest restricts flexion of the head. Maternal soft tissues are stretched more and the midwife may suspect this position if there is gaping of the vagina and dilatation of the anus, while the fetal head is barely visible. Upward moulding and caput succedaneum are evident and the baby is born face to pubis – persistent occipitoposterior (POP).

On delivery the sinciput will emerge under the symphysis and the midwife may support the head to prevent rapid expulsion of the occiput over the perineum. Management will depend on whether the midwife uses a hands-on or hands-poised method. Increased risk for perineal trauma must be anticipated in both cases.

Deep transverse arrest

If engagement occurs in the right oblique diameter of the brim, descent occurs in the right oblique diameter as a right occipitoposterior position. Descent continues to the pelvic floor and progress again depends on flexion of the head. As the head descends with a degree of flexion, the occiput begins to rotate forwards as in a long internal rotation. However, without complete flexion the occipitofrontal diameter becomes trapped in the bispinous diameter of the outlet. On vaginal examination, the sagittal suture is found in the transverse diameter usually with both fontanelles palpable. The fetal head does not advance. Medical assistance should be summoned and rotational forceps or manual rotation may be attempted. However, recent trends have ensured that most of these cases are delivered by caesarean section.

Instrumental delivery with an OP position has been shown to increase maternal morbidity.[36,37] Therefore, if instrumental delivery is deemed to be difficult, the consensus is that caesarean delivery is preferable.

Occipitoposterior labour

Care and management in the home or hospital is similar. Labour with this position has been shown to have a variety of outcomes. Vigilance on the part of the midwife is vital and any sign of prolonged labour and delay at any point should alert her to the possibility of obstructed labour and medical assistance should be sought. Monitoring progress, documented on the partogram, and detailed vaginal examinations are vital. Encouraging changes of position may offer solutions and psychological support for the mother is paramount. Aware of possible outcomes, the midwife must act as advocate for the mother, and ensure that rapid interventions are not imposed without full discussion and examination of evidence. OP presentation is still a cephalic presentation and is within the scope of midwifery practice. As with all deliveries, advance preparation for neonatal resuscitation should be made.[38]

Face presentation

Face presentation is when the area from the glabella to the undersurface of the chin lies over the cervical os. This occurs in about 1:600 cases[3] and the denominator is the mentum. The head is fully extended. The face may be a primary presentation (arising before the start of labour) or result from an OP position. The latter is called a secondary face presentation and develops during labour when a deflexed-posterior position is held up at the pelvic brim, with the contractions promoting extension of the head.

Vaginal examination

The presenting part is often high and on digital examination will feel soft and irregular. Facial features may be felt, although oedema can often distort the landmarks. The mouth and two malar prominences or orbital ridges will be felt as a triangle. Care must be taken not to damage the eyes.

Mechanism in labour

Engagement is usually in the transverse diameter of the brim, producing a right or left mentolateral position. Descent continues until the pelvic floor is reached by the mentum and rotation occurs. The mentum rotates forwards until it sits under the symphysis pubis. Descent increases extension of the face as the occiput is pushed further towards the fetal back.

After anterior rotation and descent, the chin and mouth appear at the vulva. Then the nose, eyes, brow and occiput sweep the perineum and the head delivers by flexion. The chin then rotates to the side towards which it was originally directed (restitution) and the shoulders are delivered as normal. The face will appear bruised and congested and although this may resolve within 48 hours

the establishment of breast feeding may be delayed. In extreme cases the baby may need temporary admission to the special care baby unit for support if excessive oedema compromises respiration.

Delivery

Over 50% of face presentations are not diagnosed until the second stage[39] and intervention is not warranted unless there is severe fetal distress, arrest of dilatation or arrest of descent.

The midwife can be reassured that the majority of mentoanterior positions (75% of cases) will deliver spontaneously, although the first stage is slower due to the poorly fitting presenting part. Unless the fetus is very small, delivery from the mentoposterior position will not occur. The fetal neck is shorter than the maternal sacrum and cannot stretch to fill the hollow of the sacrum. In the past it has been suggested that rotation with Kjellands forceps and delivering anteriorly may be possible, but more commonly today a caesarean section will be undertaken.[3]

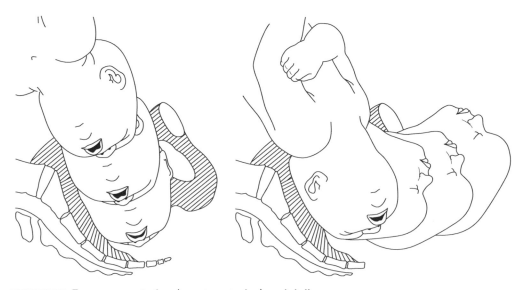

FIGURE 6.7 Face presentation (mentoanterior) and delivery

Brow presentation

This is an intermediate presentation between a 'military' attitude and a face presentation. Brow presentation occurs when the fetal head is partially extended with the brow presenting. The fetus presents with the mentovertical as the potential engaging diameter (13.5 cm). This exceeds all diameters within the pelvis. This presentation has a reported incidence of about 1:200–500.[27] The majority of cases occur without reason, although the presentation is associated with contracted pelves and an OP position.[40] If occurring as a result of an OP presentation, the brow presentation may continue to extend to a face presentation (see above) otherwise arrest of the brow occurs and labour will become obstructed.

Diagnosis

Diagnosis is difficult, with a large head palpable abdominally.

Vaginal examination

In most cases, on vaginal examination the pelvis may feel empty, although it may be possible to reach a high presenting part. The anterior fontanelle may be felt on one side of the pelvis and the orbital ridges on the other, unless they are obscured by oedema.

Labour

Caesarean section should be anticipated as vaginal delivery is rare; in most cases, brow presentation constitutes obstructed labour. However, if continued extension converts the brow to a face presentation a vaginal delivery may be possible.

Compound presentation

This occurs when a hand or a foot lie alongside the head. Unless the fetus is small they cannot both enter the pelvis together. In the majority of cases the limb withdraws as the presenting part advances. If this does not occur and the pelvis is adequate, it may be possible to push the limb back behind the head.

Possible complications of malpositions

Fetus/baby

- Hypoxia resulting from prolonged labour or cord prolapse (predisposed by a high head with an ill-fitting presenting part)
- Risk of infection if there is prolonged rupture of membranes
- Cerebral haemorrhage from unfavourable upward moulding
- Facial bruising with face presentation
- Hypothermia and hypoglycaemia if hypoxic or if resuscitation has been required.

Mother

- Prolonged labour
- Exhaustion, dehydration and ketosis
- Perineal lacerations and trauma
- Trauma from operative or instrumental delivery
- Risk of infection if prolonged rupture of membranes has taken place
- Psychological trauma.

Summary of outcomes of malposition

- Long rotation to occipitoanterior and normal OA delivery
- Short rotation to POP with face to pubis delivery

- Deep transverse arrest
- Conversion to brow presentation (may convert to face or vertex; if not, vaginal delivery unlikely)
- Conversion to face presentation (mentoanterior can deliver vaginally, mentoposterior unlikely)
- Call for medical assistance if fetal delay or arrest, or non-vertex presentation occurs
- Medical intervention for instrumental or operative delivery.

Midwifery actions

- Psychological and emotional support for the mother
- Monitor progress of labour and refer as appropriate
- Monitor well-being and position of fetus and refer as appropriate
- Prepare for neonatal resuscitation
- Keep the baby warm
- Early feeding
- Paediatric assessment
- Debrief as necessary (*see* Chapter 13).

Conclusion

Malpresentations and malpositions are often part of the birth process. Midwives should always expect the unexpected even while promoting birth as a normal physiological and psychosocial event in the life of the woman and her family. Safe practice based on sound theory is vital and such knowledge must include all aspects of the birth process. Practice, judgement and skills need to be constantly reviewed and updated.

References

1 Walkinshaw S. (2007) Breech delivery and external cephalic version. In: Grady K, Howell C, Cox C, editors. *Managing Obstetric Emergencies and Trauma: The MOET Course Manual*. London: RCOG Press. pp. 265–80.

2 Anderson GL, Irgens LM, Skranes J. (2009) Is breech presentation a risk factor for cerebral palsy? A Norwegian birth cohort study. *Dev Med Child Neurol*. 51(11): 860–5.

3 Lui DTY. (2007) Malpresentation and malpositions. In: Lui DTY, editor. *Labour Ward Manual*. 4th ed. Oxford: Churchill Livingstone.

4 Draycott T, Winter C, Crofts J, Barnfield S. (2008) *Vaginal Breech Module 9. PROMPT Practical Obstetric Multiprofessional Training*. Course Manual. London: RCOG Press. pp. 127–31.

5 Penn Z. (2006) Breech presentation. In: James D, Weiner C, Steer P, *et al.*, editors. *High Risk Pregnancy: management options*. 3rd ed. Philadelphia: Elsevier Saunders.

6 Hofmeyr GJ. (2000) Breech presentation and abnormal lie in late pregnancy. In: Enkin M, Keirse MJNC, Neilson J, *et al.*, editors. *A Guide to Effective Care in Pregnancy and Childbirth*. New York: Oxford University Press.

7 Vendittelli F, Riviere O, Crenn-Hebert C, *et al.* (2008) Is a breech presentation at term more frequent in women with a history of caesarean delivery? *Am J Obstet Gynecol*. 198(5): 521.e1–e6.

8 Rayl J, Gibson PJ, Hickok DE. (1996) A population-based case-controlled study of risk factors for breech presentation. *Am J Obstet Gynecol*. 174(1): 28–32.

9 Royal College of Obstetricians and Gynaecologists (RCOG). (2006) *External Cephalic Version (ECV) and Reducing the Incidence of Breech Presentation (Green-top 20a) and Breech Presentation, Management (Green-top 20b)*. London: RCOG Press.

10 Smith C, Crowther C, Wilkinson C, *et al.* (1999) Knee-chest postural management for breech at term: a randomised controlled trial. *Birth*. 26(2): 71–5.

11 Hofmeyr GJ, Kulier R. (2000) Cephalic version by postural management for breech presentation. (Date of most recent substantive update: 10 March 2000). *Cochrane Database Syst Rev.* 3: CD0000051.

12 Kariminia A, Chamberlain ME, Keogh J, *et al.* (2004) Randomised controlled trial of effect of hands and knees posturing on incidence of occiput posterior position at birth. *BMJ.* 328(7438): 490–3.

13 Grabowska C. (2006) Turning the breech using moxibustion. *RCM Midwives.* 9(12): 484–5.

14 Ewies A, Olah K. (2002) Moxibustion in breech version – a descriptive review. *Acupunct Med.* 20: 26–9.

15 Hofmeyr GJ, Hutton EK. (2006) External cephalic version for breech presentation before term (Cochrane Review). (Date of most recent substantive update: 18 October 2005). *Cochrane Database Syst Rev.* 1: CD000084.

16 Slome Cohain J. (2007) Turning breech babies after 34 weeks: a review. *MIDIRS Midwifery Digest.* 17(3): 373–5.

17 Cronk M. (2008) Keep your hands off the breech. *Home Birth Association of Ireland Newsletter.* 26(1): 4–6.

18 Department of Health (DH). (2007) *Maternity Matters: choice, access and continuity of care in a safe service.* London: DH Publications.

19 MIDIRS. (2008) *Where will you have your Baby?* 5th ed. Bristol: MIDIRS.

20 MIDIRS. (2008) *If your Baby is in the Breech Position, What are your Choices?* 5th ed. Bristol: MIDIRS.

21 Chinnock M, Robson S. (2007) Obstetric trainees' experience in vaginal breech delivery: implications for future practice. *Obstet Gynaecol.* 110(4): 900–3.

22 Sharma JB, Newman MR, Boutchier JE, *et al.* (1997) National audit on the practice and training in breech delivery in the UK. *Int J Gynaecol Obstet.* 59(2): 103–8.

23 Singh S, Patterson-Brown S. (2003) Malpresentations in labour. *Curr Obstet Gynaecol.* 13(5): 300–6.

24 Hannah ME, Hannah WJ, Hewson SA, *et al.* (2000) Term Breech Trial Collaborative Group, 2000. Planned caesarean section versus planned vaginal birth for breech presentation at term: a randomised multicentre trial. *Lancet.* 356: 1375–83.

25 Su M, McLeod L, Ross S, *et al.* (2003) Factors associated with adverse perinatal outcome in the term breech trial. *Am J Obstet Gynaecol.* 189: 740–5.

26 Gyte J, Frohlich J. (2001) Commentary on planned caesarean section versus planned vaginal birth for breech presentation at term: a randomised multicentre trial. *MIDIRS Midwifery Digest.* 11(1): 80–3.

27 MacKenzie I. (2006) Unstable lie, malpresentations and malpositions. In: James D, Weiner C, Steer P, *et al.*, editors. *High Risk Pregnancy: management options.* 3rd ed. Philadelphia: Elsevier Saunders.

28 Gardberg M, Stenwall O, Laakkonen E. (2004) Recurrent persistent occipito-posterior position in subsequent deliveries. *BJOG.* 111(2): 170–1.

29 Gardberg M, Laakkonen ES, Levaara M. (1998) Intrapartum sonography and persistent occiput posterior position: a study of 408 deliveries. *Obstet Gynecol.* 91(5/1): 746–9.

30 Sutton J. (2000) Occipito-posterior positioning and some ideas about how to change it. *Pract Midwife.* 3(6): 20–2.

31 Walmsley K. (2000) Managing the occipitoposterior labour. *MIDIRS Midwifery Digest.* 10(1): 61–2.

32 Hunter S, Hofmeyr GJ, Kulier R. (2007) Hands and knees posture in late pregnancy or labour for fetal malposition (lateral or posterior). Cochrane *Database Syst Rev.* 4: CD001063.

33 El Halta V. (1996) Posterior labor – a pain in the back! Its prevention and cure. *Clarion.* 11(1): 6–7, 12–13.

34 Sinclair C. (2004) *A Midwife's Handbook.* St Louis: Saunders.

35 Reichman O, Gdansky E, Latinsky B, *et al.* (2008) Digital rotation from occipito-posterior to occipito-anterior decreases the need for cesarean section. *Eur J Obstet Gynecol Reprod Biol.* 136(1): 25–8.

36 Benavides L, Wu JM, Hundley AF. (2005) The impact of occiput posterior

fetal head position on the risk of anal sphincter injury in forceps-assisted vaginal deliveries. *Am J Obstet Gynecol.* **192**(5): 1702–6.

37 Wu JM, Williams KS, Hundley AF. (2005) Occiput posterior fetal head position increases the risk of anal sphincter injury in vacuum-assisted deliveries. *Am J Obstet Gynecol.* **193**(2): 525–9.

38 Cheng YW, Shaffer BL, Caughey AB. (2006) The association between persistent occiput posterior position and neonatal outcomes. *Obstet Gynaecol.* **107**(4): 837–44.

39 Bhal PS, Davies NJ, Chung T. (1998) A population study of face and brow presentation. *J Obstet Gynaecol.* **18**(3): 231–5.

40 Bashiri A, Burnstein E, Bar-David J. (2008) Face and brow presentation: independent risk factors. *J Matern Fetal Neonatal Med.* **21**(6): 357–60.

CHAPTER 7

Umbilical cord prolapse

Caroline Squire

Cord prolapse is defined as prolapse of the umbilical cord alongside (occult) or past the presenting part in the presence of ruptured membranes[1] (*see* Figure 7.1). Cord presentation occurs without the presence of ruptured membranes.

Cord prolapse is an obstetric emergency with a reported incidence varying between 0.1% and 0.6% of all births, but this increases to a little above 1%

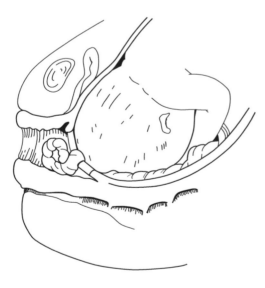

in breech presentations.[2,3] Murphy and MacKenzie[4] examined the management of cord prolapse and occurrence of morbidity and mortality in a retrospective study of 132 babies born after identification of cord prolapse. They concluded that it occurred at a relatively stable rate irrespective of changes in obstetric practices,[5] and that the fetal outcome was not as poor as might be expected, mortality predominantly being attributable to congenital anomalies and prematurity rather than birth asphyxia. In the last few years, however, there has been a significant increase in the delivery of breech babies by caesarean section and this has contributed to a slight reduction in the incidence of cord prolapse.[6]

Cord prolapse is an independent risk factor for perinatal death[3] and, one large study found a perinatal mortality rate of 91:1000.[4] The interval between diagnosis and delivery is significantly related to stillbirth and neonatal death so that if cord prolapse occurs outside the hospital maternity unit, the prognosis is worse.[7] Asphyxia may also result in hypoxic-ischaemic encephalopathy and cerebral palsy. It is thought that this is most likely to be caused by cord compression and umbilical arterial vasospasm preventing venous and arterial blood flow to and from the fetus.[8]

Risk factors

The principle to remember is that whenever there is room for the cord to slip into the pelvis there is the potential for cord presentation or cord prolapse (*see* Table 7.1). In addition, there is an increased risk associated with some procedures such as artificial rupture of membranes, external cephalic version, stabilising induction of labour, applying fetal scalp electrode and rotational instrumental delivery.[7]

Diagnosis

Cord presentation

This may be diagnosed on vaginal examination when the cord is felt behind intact membranes. It may also be suspected when the midwife detects abnormalities in the fetal heart rate.

Cord prolapse

Umbilical cord prolapse is diagnosed when the cord can be seen externally or palpated in the vagina or alongside the presenting part by the midwife. It may also be suspected when severe, recurrent variable decelerations or bradycardia occur in the fetal heart rate which does not respond to change in maternal position. Once diagnosed, the objective is to maintain the fetal circulation by preventing cord compression and expedite delivery. If the incident occurs at a home birth, transfer by ambulance should be as swift as possible and the maternity unit should be notified of what is happening prior to arrival. A situation such as this emphasises the importance of having two midwives present at home births. Perinatal mortality is increased by more than ten-fold when cord prolapse occurs outside the hospital as is neonatal morbidity.[8]

TABLE 7.1 Risk factors for cord prolapse[8]

General	Procedure related
Multiparity	Artificial rupture of membranes
Low birth weight, less than 2.5 kg	Vaginal manipulation of fetus with ruptured membranes
Prematurity: less than 37 weeks	External cephalic version (during procedure)
Fetal congenital anomalies	Internal podalic version
Breech presentation	Stabilising induction of labour
Transverse, oblique and unstable lie	Insertion of uterine pressure transducer
Second twin	
Polyhydramnios	
Unengaged presenting part	
Low-lying placenta; other abnormal placentation	

Management

The management of cord prolapse is one of the delivery suite guidelines mandated by the Clinical Negligence Scheme for Trusts (CNST), Welsh Pool Risk and Clinical Negligence and Other Risks Scheme (CNORIS) maternity standards in England, Wales and Scotland, respectively.[8] It must be remembered that this emergency situation will frighten the mother and her partner, and midwives need to communicate sensitively and explicitly so that the parents understand the gravity of the situation without losing control. Accurate and concurrent record keeping is essential as is the recording of the fetal heart until delivery is imminent.

Draycott *et al.*[7] offer an outline for the management of cord prolapse as follows (*see* Figure 7.2).

Cord presentation

In the case of cord presentation diagnosed on vaginal examination, the membranes should be left intact and the mother helped into a position that will relieve cord compression (*see* Figures 7.3 and 7.4).

Cord prolapse

1 Manual elevation of the presenting part above the pelvic inlet to relieve cord compression. This is accomplished by the midwife inserting two fingers onto the presenting part and applying pressure.

2 An all-fours position, with buttocks raised and with manual elevation of the presenting part above the pelvic brim (*see* Figure 7.3) or exaggerated Sims' position (*see* Figure 7.4) to elevate the woman's buttocks and relieve pressure on the umbilical cord. The latter is the more appropriate position for transfer by ambulance.

3 If the umbilical cord has prolapsed out of the body, there is some controversy as to whether or not to replace it in the vagina.[8] It is suggested that exposure to the cold air may cause

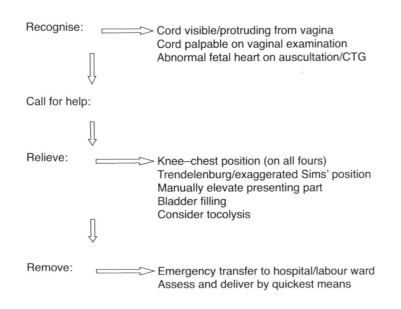

Recognise: ⟹ Cord visible/protruding from vagina
Cord palpable on vaginal examination
Abnormal fetal heart on auscultation/CTG

Call for help:

Relieve: ⟹ Knee–chest position (on all fours)
Trendelenburg/exaggerated Sims' position
Manually elevate presenting part
Bladder filling
Consider tocolysis

Remove: ⟹ Emergency transfer to hospital/labour ward
Assess and deliver by quickest means

FIGURE 7.2 Management of cord prolapse

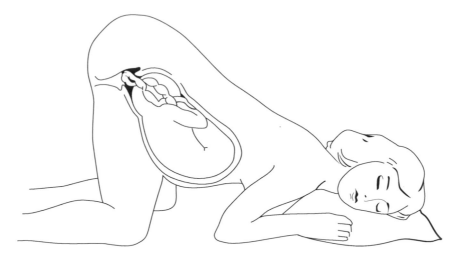

FIGURE 7.3 All-fours position with buttocks raised

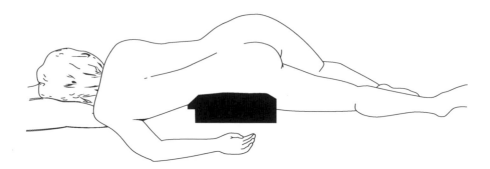

FIGURE 7.4 Exaggerated Sims' position

vasoconstriction, but handling the cord may also have this effect.

4 Fill the maternal bladder with 400–700 ml of saline solution. This may relieve cord compression and also inhibit uterine contractions, thus decreasing pressure on the cord.[9–11] A 16G Foley catheter and standard giving set are used to rapidly fill the bladder.[12]

5 Amnioinfusion of saline or Ringers lactate solution has been described for cord compression in labour but is not common practice. In a systematic review, Hofmeyr[13] found amnioinfusion to be useful in reducing the occurrence of variable fetal heart rate decelerations, improving short-term measures of neonatal outcome, and lowering the use of caesarean section, mainly for 'fetal distress' diagnosed by fetal heart rate monitoring alone. He further states in his conclusion, however, that the trials reviewed were too small to assess maternal effect.

If the cervix is fully dilated and the presenting part is engaged, vaginal delivery may be appropriate through maternal effort or with ventouse or forceps. If vaginal delivery is not possible, emergency caesarean section should be performed as soon as possible with prior emptying of the maternal bladder.[9,14,15]

Once the diagnosis of umbilical cord prolapse is made, rapid delivery of the baby is vital. However, in a retrospective review of 65 cases of umbilical cord prolapse it was postulated that the cases of neonatal asphyxia associated with cord prolapse may have been aggravated by factors other than time.[16] It was speculated that the degree of cord compression and the amount of amniotic fluid could affect neonatal outcome.

It may be that time spent resuscitating the fetus *in utero* by maternal position changes, inserting a urinary catheter and filling the bladder or administering tocolysis may be beneficial to the fetus and lead to a lower incidence of neonatal asphyxia. The study also found that occult cord prolapse was associated with less perinatal morbidity when compared to frank prolapse.[16]

Multiprofessional training is now common in maternity units but simulated training for umbilical cord prolapse is less common. Many units practise simulated emergencies in terms of shoulder dystocia, postpartum haemorrhage, neonatal and maternal resuscitation, but umbilical cord prolapse is often omitted. However, Siassakos *et al.*[17] published a retrospective cohort study to determine whether the introduction of multiprofessional simulation training was associated with improvements in the management of cord prolapse, in particular the diagnosis–delivery interval. They reviewed all cases of cord prolapse with informative case records – 34 pre-training and 28 post-training. After training, they found that there was a statistically significant reduction in the median diagnosis – delivery interval and a statistically significant increase in the proportion of births by caesarean section. They concluded that annual training was associated with improved management of cord prolapse but future studies were needed to see if this translated into better outcomes for babies and their mothers.

The importance of record keeping that is factual, contemporaneous and detailed cannot be overemphasised. In a retrospective audit to investigate the standards of practice in the management of cord prolapse in one maternity unit, the record keeping was not found to contain poor documentation in terms of information concerning manoeuvres to relieve pressure on the umbilical cord, but was poor concerning communication with the woman and her partner.[18]

Finally, Qureshi, Taylor and Tomlinson[19] published a retrospective review to assess current practice and outcomes for women who experienced cord prolapse at their birth. They found that of the 15 273 births that occurred between March 1999 and February 2003, 19 cases of cord prolapse were identified: 15 cases occurred on the delivery suite, three on the antenatal ward and one at home; four cases occurred in a twin, five in fetuses in breech presentation, and one in a fetus in a transverse lie. All women were delivered by emergency caesarean section. They reported a rate of 1.2:1000. Some of their patients had their bladder filled with 400–700 ml of saline solution to elevate the presenting part and also, thereby, having a tocolytic effect on the uterus. Their mean diagnosis to delivery time was 16 minutes. Three of the

19 newborns had Apgar scores of less than 7 at five minutes and two required admission to the special care baby unit. However, importantly, all of the newborns fared well in the end and did not suffer neurological sequelae.

Checklist for midwives

- If at home, call for immediate transfer by ambulance, position the woman appropriately, relieve pressure digitally and consider filling her bladder.
- In hospital: call for help – coordinating midwife; senior obstetrician, senior paediatrician, senior anaesthetist.
- Communicate with the woman and birth partner.
- Relieve cord compression to enable fetal oxygenation: maternal position (all fours, buttocks raised or exaggerated Sims'); relieve pressure digitally from the umbilical cord.
- Record keeping.
- Reflect on experience with peers and/or supervisor of midwives.
- Consider risk management issues.
- Help parents debrief if appropriate (*see* Chapter 13).

References

1 Johanson R, Cox C. (1999) Cord prolapse. In: Cox C, Grady K, editors. *Managing Obstetric Emergencies*. Oxford: Bios Scientific Publishers.
2 Lin M. (2006) Umbilical cord prolapse. *Obstet Gynecol Surv.* **61**: 269–77.
3 Kahana B, Sheiner E, Levy A, Lazer S, Mazor M. (2004) Umbilical cord prolapse and perinatal outcomes. *Int J Gynnaecol Obstet.* **84**: 127–32.
4 Murphy DJ, MacKenzie IZ. (1995) The mortality and morbidity associated with umbilical cord prolapse. *Br J Obstet Gynaecol.* **102**: 826–30.
5 Roberts WE, Martin RW, Roach HH, *et al.* (1997) Are obstetric interventions such as cervical ripening, induction of labor, amnioinfusion or amniotomy associated with umbilical cord prolapse? *Am J Obstet Gynecol.* **176**(6): 1181–5.
6 Nizard J, Cromi A, Molendijk H, Arabin B. (2005) Neonatal outcome following prolonged umbilical cord prolapse in preterm premature rupture of membranes *Br J Obstet Gynaecol.* **112**: 833–6.
7 Draycott T, Winter C, Crofts J, Barnsfield S, editors (2008) *PROMPT: Practical Obstetric Multiprofessional Training.* Course Manual. London: RCOG Press.
8 Royal College of Obstetricians and Gynaecologists (RCOG). (2008) Umbilical Cord Prolapse: Green-top Guideline No. 50. Available at: www.rcog.org.uk (accessed 19 July 2009).
9 Johanson R, Cox C. (1999) Cord prolapse. In: Cox C, Grady K, editors. *Managing Obstetric Emergencies*. Oxford: Bios Scientific Publishers.
10 McGeown P. (2001) Practice recommendations for obstetric emergencies. *Br J Midwif.* **9**(2): 71–3.
11 Runnebaum IB, Katz M. (1999) Intrauterine resuscitation by rapid urinary bladder instillation in a case of occult prolapse of an excessively long umbilical cord. *Eur J Obstet Gynecol Repro Biol.* **84**(1): 101–2.
12 Houghton G. (2006) Bladder filling: an effective technique for managing cord prolapse. *Br J Midwif.* **14**(2): 88–90.
13 Hofmeyr G, Xu H. (2009) Amnioinfusion for meconium-stained liquor in labour. *Cochrane Database Syst Rev.* 1: CD000014.
14 Usta IM, Mercer BM, Sibai BM. (1999) Current obstetrical practice and umbilical cord prolapse. *Am J Perinatol.* **16**(9): 479–84.
15 Critchlow CW, Leet TL, Benedetti TJ, Daling JR. (1994) Risk factors and infant outcomes associated with umbilical cord prolapse: a population-based case-control study among births in Washington State. *Am J Obstet Gynecol.* **170**: 613–18.

16 Prabulos A-M, Philipson EH. (1998) Umbilical cord prolapse: is the time from diagnosis to delivery critical? *J Reprod Med.* **43**: 129–32.

17 Siassakos D, Hasafa Z, Sibanda T, *et al.* (2009) Retrospective cohort study of diagnosis-delivery interval with umbilical cord prolapse: the effect of team training. *BJOG.* **116**(8): 1089–96.

18 Rogers C, Schiavone N. (2008) Cord prolapse audit: recognition, management and outcome. *Br J Midwif.* **16**(5): 315–18.

19 Quereshi NS, Taylor DJ, Tomlinson AJ. (2004) Brief communication: umbilical cord prolapse. *Int J Gynecol Obstet.* **86**: 29–30.

CHAPTER 8

Uterine rupture and uterine inversion

Maureen Boyle

Uterine rupture

A full or complete uterine rupture is defined as a tear through the full thickness of the myometrium and the overlaying peritoneum, with or without the expulsion of the fetus into the abdominal cavity. A complete uterine rupture is a very serious complication of labour that can lead to fetal death and contributes to maternal morbidity and mortality. It may also occur during pregnancy, usually after 32 weeks' gestation and particularly in the presence of a classical (longitudinal) uterine scar. A partial or incomplete rupture does not extend through the full thickness of the uterus and may, in a scarred uterus, involve scar dehiscence. It usually presents with less acute symptoms, or may be discovered accidentally.

Although a uterine rupture can happen spontaneously in those with no risk factors, this is rare. There are many risk factors identified that may predispose to a uterine rupture, and knowledge of them may help a midwife to anticipate or interpret signs and symptoms correctly, if the situation should occur.

The incidence of uterine rupture varies widely throughout the literature. The risk of uterine rupture increases in women who have had a previous caesarean section, and prior uterine surgery is considered to be the main cause for rupture in the developed world.[1] It has been suggested that rates for uterine rupture in the USA have significantly reduced over the past 20 years as the number of women undertaking vaginal birth after caesarean (VBAC) has fallen.[2] Therefore contemporary American figures demonstrate about 50% of uterine ruptures happening with no history of caesarean section. However, the majority of those without previous caesarean section were receiving oxytocin and/or prostaglandins. The drop in the overall rate may also have to do with the decrease in practices such as internal podalic version, fundal pressure and rotational forceps.

In the UK the incidence of uterine rupture is quoted as 5.2 per 1000 VBAC, with a perinatal death rate of 1 per 2000 and maternal death rate rare at <1:10 000.[3] A rupture of an unscarred uterus is quoted as approximately 1:8000–15 000.[4]

In less developed countries the rate

of uterine rupture is estimated at 1%[1] presumably because of a high rate of unrelieved obstructed labour.[5]

Risk/predisposing factors

Although much of the literature focuses on uterine rupture following previous caesarean section, other factors have been identified (see Box 8.1).

BOX 8.1 Risk/predisposing factors for uterine rupture[4,6–12]

- Grandmultiparity
- Previous uterine surgery (including minimally invasive procedures)
- Previous uterine rupture
- Abnormal placentation
- Some medical conditions
- Pharmacological induction/ augmentation of labour
- Abdominal trauma (e.g. violence)
- Interventional obstetric procedures (e.g. internal podalic version, assisted breech)
- Obstructed labour
- Abnormal uterus.

Parity

Traditional teaching in midwifery and obstetrics was that 'primips don't rupture'. However, although rare, a number of cases in primigravid women have been reported.[4]

A Dutch study of multiparous women with uterine rupture demonstrated a perinatal mortality rate of 11.7%.[7] In a study of primigravid women with uterine rupture, a perinatal mortality rate of 26% was identified.[4] There was also a 20% hysterectomy rate in the primigravida study[4] vs. 4% in the study of multiparous women.[7] The suggestion was cited that the diagnosis and therefore treatment for multiparous women may be reached more speedily as suspicion is higher. However, it is assumed that many of the multiparous women will have ruptured through a scar, which may be less catastrophic as scarred tissue is less vascular than unscarred tissue, and in addition it was presumably easier to repair a previous incision than a primary rupture. Nevertheless, it is a salutary lesson that a primiparous woman may have a uterine rupture, and the consequences may be tragic.

Previous caesarean section

It is hard to exactly quantify the risk of a previous caesarean section scar rupture, as the literature reports vary widely. The RCOG considers women should be informed that VBAC carries a risk of uterine rupture of 22–74:10 000[13] and the National Institute for Health and Clinical Excellence (NICE) state that women should be informed that uterine rupture during VBAC is a very rare complication but is increased in women planning vaginal birth.[14] However, when discussing a VBAC with a woman, it would be wise to consider her individual factors. Risk factors from previous caesarean sections can be assessed in pregnancy – Shipp et al.[15] has developed a numerical score using several of the more common risk factors.

- **Previous classical (longitudinal) incision:** Uterine rupture is less common when any scar from a previous caesarean section is in the lower segment because this is the portion of the uterus that does not contract. The incidence of uterine rupture is greater in women who have had a classic uterine incision.[3] A previous classical incision also holds an increased risk for antenatal uterine rupture.

- **Interpregnancy interval:** It is suggested that there is more risk of a uterine rupture if the time interval between labour and the previous caesarean section is less than 18 months.[16] One large study identified that the risk of uterine rupture was 4.8% with an interpregnancy interval of 5–12 months, which then dropped to 0.9% with an interval of more than 36 months.[17]
- **Previous labour or vaginal delivery:** Labour before the primary caesarean section appears to decrease the rate of rupture in subsequent VBACs.[18] There also appears to be a protective effect of prior vaginal delivery whether it was before or after the caesarean section.[19]
- **The number of previous caesarean sections:** The number of previous caesarean sections appears to influence the risk of uterine rupture[20] but the number is not consistent in the literature. Previous preterm caesarean section may also be a predisposing factor for uterine rupture,[20] although of course the type of incision used would also have an influence on this.
- **Previous wound closure:** Although some research has demonstrated that single layer closure is associated with an increased risk of rupture,[17] there still appears to be controversy over whether to use single or double layer closure to reduce the risk of uterine rupture.[13]
- **Previous wound healing:** Prolonged healing (with or without infection) of the scar may result in a scar that may be more easily disrupted.[18]

Previous surgical procedure

It would appear that any previous surgical procedure affecting the uterus, such as myomectomy, excision of endometriosis implants and dilatation and curettage (D&C) can predispose to a spontaneous uterine rupture.[4,8] Although previously it was considered that only full-thickness uterine scars were a risk factor for uterine rupture, there is now increasing evidence from minimally invasive surgeries such as laparascopy.[8]

Abnormal placentation

A scarred uterus with placenta percreta may lead to rupture.[9,21] In a study of 120 636 pregnancies there were seven spontaneous ruptures in women with previous caesarean sections but before labour commenced. Six were with abnormal placentation.[21] Other associations were short interpregnancy intervals and past uterine rupture.[22]

Medical conditions

Hypertension and pre-eclampsia have been over-represented in some studies[10] and it is considered these conditions may contribute a propensity to rupture.

There is some evidence that women who experienced intrapartum and postpartum pyrexia during their prior caesarean birth had increased risk of uterine rupture in the next pregnancy.[11]

Pharmacological induction/ augmentation: oxytocin and/or prostaglandins

A two- to three-fold increased risk of uterine rupture in induced and/or augmented labours compared with spontaneous labours has been demonstrated.[13] An induction of labour, even after a previous vaginal delivery, can double the risk of uterine rupture.[23]

It has been suggested that uterine rupture may occur in a VBAC at a rate of 0.7%–0.98%, but in a VBAC with induction the rate could be 2%–3%.[24] Oxytocin is used for induction/augmentation with a scarred uterus and there is no doubt that some women will achieve a VBAC because of its effect. However, as would be expected, a higher dose has been found to increase the risk of rupture,[25] although even reduced doses are also associated with uterine rupture.[26] A survey of obstetric consultants in south-west England found most would use prostaglandins and oxytocin for a woman in a VBAC labour.[26]

Abdominal trauma

Abdominal trauma from whatever cause, for example accidental injury (such as a motor vehicle accident), or domestic violence,[27] has been demonstrated to cause uterine rupture. Uterine rupture can also be caused by obstetric techniques such as manipulation during pregnancy or labour to correct an unstable lie or malpresentation (e.g. external cephalic or internal podalic versions), manual removal of the placenta, shoulder dystocia and use of fundal pressure in the second stage of labour.

Signs and symptoms

Signs and symptoms vary greatly and depend on the stage of labour and degree of rupture or dehiscence, as well as the site of rupture (the lower segment is more common in labour, although the posterior fundus is considered to be the weakest part of the uterus). It should be noted that the signs and symptoms overlap significantly with those of a concealed abruption,[4] and this diagnosis should also be considered.

Fetal heart rate abnormalities

The earliest sign of uterine rupture is frequently an abnormal fetal heart rate pattern – which is why many hospital protocols together with the RCOG recommend continuous CTGs during a VBAC labour.[13] Abnormal patterns are suggested to be present in 55%–87% of uterine ruptures.[28]

Slowing down or cessation of contractions

The slowing down or abrupt cessation of contractions is often a clear sign that there is a problem with the labour. Matsuo et al.[29] describe a 'staircase sign', where the contraction pattern on a CTG is seen to gradually reduce before a sudden onset of prolonged fetal bradycardia. However, internal monitoring demonstrated an increase in uterine resting tone – a sign that a midwife may identify with her hand.

The classical signs of loss of contractions followed by fetal bradycardia are also demonstrated in both scarred and unscarred uteri.[29]

Pain

Severe abdominal pain, especially if persisting between contractions[13] should lead to suspicion of uterine rupture. The pain is often of sudden onset. In a scarred uterus, tenderness may be evident before actual rupture takes place. Chest pain or shoulder tip pain has also been described.[13]

Palpation

On abdominal palpation Bandl's (retraction) ring may be palpable and the lower segment may feel distended. Palpation is usually very painful for the woman.[5] Following complete rupture fetal parts can be felt in the abdomen.

Maternal vital signs

Maternal shock may be the first sign of uterine rupture – the degree is dependent on the extent of the rupture. This may involve maternal tachycardia, hypovolaemic shock, hypotension, breathlessness and collapse.[8,13] However, although the woman can collapse (particularly if the tear goes into the broad ligament vessels) the maternal condition is usually observed to deteriorate progressively.[5]

Bleeding

Vaginal bleeding is rare as it is usually hidden behind the presenting part. If rupture occurs during a vaginal delivery (and the risk is increased with instrumental delivery) the condition may present with a postpartum haemorrhage (PPH).[5]

Haematuria is often present (and may be the first sign, especially if a woman is catheterised) because the bladder may be adherent to a previous uterine scar.

Incomplete rupture

There may be no signs and symptoms; however, if present their onset is gradual. Labour may slow down, especially in primigravid women. An incomplete rupture may only be diagnosed retrospectively at caesarean section or at laparotomy investigation for postpartum haemorrhage.

Management

There has been some suggestion that an antenatal ultrasound assessment of the thickness of the lower segment in those with previous caesarean section may predict those at increased risk of scar dehiscence and/or rupture,[30] but more research needs to be undertaken before this can be included in routine practice.[31]

Management in hospital

- Summon urgent help. As with all acute obstetric emergencies this should include a senior obstetrician and an obstetric anaesthetist.
- Stop oxytocin infusion if it is being used.
- Resuscitate and treat the shock, including cannulation, fluid administration, constant monitoring of vital signs (*see* Chapter 2 for treatment and management of shock).
- Obtain consents and prepare for surgical delivery or laparotomy.

Management at home

- Early recognition of signs and symptoms is essential.
- Summon urgent help. Call paramedics and arrange for immediate ambulance transfer into hospital. Alert the nearest consultant-led maternity unit.
- Resuscitate and treat shock while awaiting paramedic assistance (*see* Chapter 2).

Outcome

Uterine repair of a rupture is usually possible but if not – and this is more common when there is a spontaneous rupture of an unscarred uterus – hysterectomy may be necessary.[5] If the rupture is particularly large, or the woman's condition is threatened, a hysterectomy may be a life-saving operation.[32]

The outcome of the next pregnancy – or indeed whether another pregnancy is recommended – will depend on where the rupture was located.[8] A planned caesarean section for the next pregnancy may be suggested.[5]

Conclusion

As women with pre-existing uterine scars are the group most at risk of uterine rupture, careful consideration must be given when planning the management of future pregnancies and labours. However, the long held guiding principle of 'once a caesarean, always a caesarean' is no longer the accepted mantra in most maternity units.

Adherence to safe guiding principles should allow the majority of women who choose vaginal birth after a previous caesarean to deliver with minimal risk. However, these women should be carefully selected. Information about the previous caesarean section, including pre-operative events and postoperative recovery, should be carefully scrutinised. The RCOG recommends that the women's views and wishes should be borne in mind when making plans for delivery.[13]

Labour and vaginal delivery following previous caesarean section can therefore be recommended providing the following points apply.

- There has been early counselling and education on the signs and symptoms of uterine scar separation. This will facilitate an informed decision and choice on the part of the pregnant woman with regard to the place and mode of delivery.
- Sufficient obstetric and anaesthetic backup is readily available in the maternity unit.
- Women with risk factors have been identified. This group should have an agreed, documented plan of management for labour and delivery. This should include a readiness to proceed to emergency caesarean section in the event of prolonged labour, fetal distress or scar pain, any or all of which may indicate imminent scar dehiscence or uterine rupture.

Uterine inversion

Uterine inversion is a rare but life-threatening complication of the third stage of labour and is classified by time and severity. The uterus can be described as inverted when the fundus has prolapsed into the body of the uterus and beyond. When this occurs immediate action must be taken to prevent maternal morbidity and mortality.

Uterine inversion has been cited as occurring at a rate of anywhere from 1:2000 to 1:6400.[33] The widespread variation in this rate may be dependent on third-stage management and the level of reporting.[12]

- **Acute uterine inversion**: This can occur during the third stage, when the placenta may or may not be attached, and up to 24 hours after delivery of the baby. It can be associated with cervical constriction and/or a cervical contraction ring (a contraction ring is a spasm – constriction – of the circular uterine muscles, usually occurring at the junction of the lower and upper uterine segments), which will impede replacement of the uterus.
- **Subacute inversion**: This occurs from 24 hours after delivery up to 28 days postpartum. A cervical contraction ring is usually present.
- **Chronic inversion**: This occurs after 28 days.

Severity

Severity is determined by degrees:[5,34]
- **First degree (incomplete)**: The fundus extends to, but not beyond, the cervix.
- **Second degree**: The fundus protrudes through the cervix into the vagina.
- **Third degree**: The fundus extends to the perineum. If the fundus, cervix

and vagina are visible this constitutes a uterine prolapse.

Aetiology

Many risk factors/causes of uterine inversion have been identified (*see* Box 8.2). However, in up to 50% of cases no risk factors can be identified, and no mismanagement of the third stage is evident.[35] Therefore a uterine inversion can be considered to be largely unpredictable.

BOX 8.2 Predisposing factors/causes of uterine inversion[5,12,35,36]

■ Mismanagement of the third stage
■ Increased uterine pressure
■ Overstretched uterus
■ Primigravida
■ Grandmultigravida
■ Fundal position of the placenta
■ Short umbilical cord
■ Abnormality of the placenta (e.g. morbidly adherent placenta)
■ Congenital anomalies of the uterus (e.g. bicornuate uterus)
■ Gravitational weight of an intrauterine mass (e.g. fibroids)
■ Connective tissue disorders.

Uterine inversion can be iatrogenic, caused by mismanagement of the third stage of labour, including:

• early and excessive controlled cord traction (CCT) before signs of placental separation
• controlled cord traction when the uterus is relaxed
• the use of fundal pressure with or without cord traction.

CCT on a relaxed uterus is the most common cause,[5] and this needs to act as a reminder to midwives of the dangers of mixing active and physiological third-stage management. The high rate of uterine inversion in developing countries is considered to be due to both the absence of active management of the third stage, plus the use of untrained birth attendants who lack the ability to safely manage a physiological third stage.[35]

However, when accurately done, active management of the third stage is considered to have decreased the incidence of uterine inversion fourfold,[37] and some clinicians[35] suggest that an increased rate of inversions should be expected in the UK if physiological management of the third stage becomes more common with the increase in community deliveries.

Uterine inversion can also occur spontaneously after rapid decompression of an overstretched uterus, as with the delivery of a macrosomic baby or twins or, rarely, following increased intra-abdominal pressure when the uterus can be forced down and out as a result of coughing, vomiting or pushing.[38]

An adherent placenta is associated with a thin relaxed myometrium, prone to inversion.[5] It is worth noting that as caesarean sections and an associated placenta accreta in the next pregnancy become more common, VBACs may become a risk category, albeit carrying only a minimal risk.

Signs and symptoms

There are two cardinal signs of uterine inversion, those of shock and pain:

• **Shock**: Signs of shock are usually sudden, profound and may be disproportionate to the amount of blood loss and degree of inversion. It occurs in response to neurogenic stimuli and hypovolaemia. Bleeding may or may not be present depending on whether the placenta is attached to the uterine wall, although the majority of women (94%) may present with haemorrhage.[35,38]

- **Pain:** Pain is characteristically severe, low abdominal and accompanied by a bearing-down sensation. It is caused by traction on the infundibulopelvic ligaments, round ligaments and the ovaries.[39]

In subacute and chronic inversion, the signs and symptoms may be less dramatic and are classically characterised by urinary retention, prolonged heavy lochia and a low pelvic 'dragging' sensation.[39]

Diagnosis

Uterine inversion is not common, but a high level of suspicion is necessary as it can be a life-threatening obstetric emergency.[38] The clinical presentation and diagnosis of uterine inversion is dependent on the classification of time and severity.

A first-degree inversion may be missed as the fundus will not be visible at the introitus or palpable at the cervix and there may be no specific signs and symptoms. However, an indentation may be palpable at the fundus. Further diagnostic tools may be necessary for a firm diagnosis, such as ultrasound or magnetic resonance imaging (MRI).

Both second and third-degree inversions will usually present with unmissable signs and symptoms as described above. With a second- and third-degree inversion, the uterus is not palpable in the abdomen and on vaginal examination the inverted fundus will be felt in the vagina or be visible at the introitus. The placenta may or may not be attached. A second or third-degree inversion requires an urgent response.[12]

Differential diagnoses

As shock is a cardinal sign, it is necessary to exclude a differential diagnosis of pulmonary or amniotic fluid embolism, myocardial infarction and uterine rupture. A prompt vaginal examination will confirm the presence of a uterine inversion and it is important to act quickly to minimise maternal morbidity and mortality. If treatment is delayed the uterus can become oedematous and congested. Delay also allows the formation of a contraction ring, which will impede replacement of the inverted fundus.

Management

Evidence and research-based protocols for the management of the third stage of labour should be in place in all units. All midwives should be familiar with both the active and physiological (expectant) management of the third stage of labour. Management of acute second and third-degree inversion in both hospital and home settings is discussed below.

Immediate management in hospital

Assistance: As with all acute obstetric emergencies, help must be urgently summoned. This should include a senior obstetrician and an obstetric anaesthetist.

The following three points should be done simultaneously, as replacement of the uterus is considered the quickest way to treat neurogenic shock:[35]

1 Resuscitation and treatment of shock (*see* Chapter 2 for treatment and management of shock).

2 Stop any oxytocin infusion: once inversion is recognised, all oxytocic agents should be withheld until correction has been established.

3 The aim of management is to replace the uterus as soon as possible. This

needs to be done before the development of a contraction ring.

Replacement of the uterus

Whether the placenta has separated or not, an attempt should be made to return the uterus to the vagina if it has prolapsed outside the introitus. Although it may appear easier to replace a smaller mass, **no attempt should be made to manually remove the placenta if it has not separated.** Removing the placenta will exacerbate shock and cause haemorrhage.[33,36,40] The attached placenta prevents bleeding because the uterine sinuses are not exposed.

Manual repositioning of the uterus

If the uterine fundus can be felt in the vagina or is visible, the uterus should be replaced. The preferred method is *Johnson's manoeuvre*.[35,41] The midwife inserts her hand into the vagina and the fundus is cupped in the palm of the hand. Pressure is exerted back up and along the long axis of the vagina with pressure directed towards the umbilicus until the uterus is back in the vagina. When feeding the uterus back through the cervix, it is important to reposition the last section of the uterus that inverted first to prevent overlapping tissue at the cervix, which would further compound oedema and congestion. This position needs to be held for several minutes or until a firm contraction occurs to ensure that the uterus remains in the pelvis. If replacement takes place before oedema of the uterus and a contraction ring develops, it should be successful.[35] Intravenous oxytocics should then be given to maintain uterine contraction, according to unit protocol. This enables the cervix to reform.

In some cases medication may be given to enable myometrial relaxation and perhaps prevent/relax a contraction ring. Most commonly used are magnesium sulphate, ritodrine, terbutaline or nitroglycerin.[33]

Following successful replacement of the uterus, manual removal of the placenta is usually done in theatre under general anaesthetic because of the risk of postpartum haemorrhage.

O'Sullivan's hydrostatic method

Hydrostatic pressure[42] involves bags of warmed fluid (e.g. normal saline/sterile water) hung above the level of the patient and allowed to flow, via tubing, into the posterior vagina. The pressure of the water, held in place by the clinician's hands, results in correction of the inversion. A modification of this method describes using a ventouse silicone cup, positioned just inside the vagina, with tubing connecting it to the fluid[33] (thus enabling a better 'seal').

If immediate replacement is not possible, the woman's condition should be stabilised and general anaesthetic administered. Manual replacement may then be possible and, if not, surgical intervention via a laparotomy will be required. If a laparotomy is undertaken, assistance may still be necessary to push the uterus through the vagina.[40]

Immediate management at home

Removal of the placenta: It is vital that no attempt should be made to remove the placenta for reasons stated above.

- **Assistance:** Call paramedics and arrange for immediate ambulance transfer into hospital. Alert the nearest consultant-led maternity unit. While awaiting paramedic assistance carry out the following procedures.

- **Resuscitation and treatment of shock:** *See* Chapter 2 for the treatment and management of shock. Even if the woman does not manifest severe symptoms, at a minimum intravenous access should be achieved.
- **Replacement of the uterus:** Immediate replacement of the uterus, using the Johnson's manoeuvre described above, should be attempted. If this is unsuccessful, and the uterus is inverted outside the vulva, an attempt should be made to return it to the vagina to prevent further shock and reduce maternal morbidity. If this is not possible, the uterus can be wrapped in sterile gauze soaked in warm saline or water. The use of a plastic bag over the top may help to retain heat and moisture. This can all be wrapped in a towel to maintain moisture and warmth and possibly delay the onset of shock. The plastic bag may also prevent the towel adhering to the uterus.

Ongoing management

Antibiotic cover is usual. Early assessment of anaemia may also be necessary.

A postnatal check by the consultant obstetrician should be undertaken, to ensure this condition is not chronic. A physiotherapy referral is often made. The woman may need counselling concerning the likelihood of recurrence in her next labour, and discussion should take place about the mode of delivery for any future pregnancies.

Early debriefing may be useful for the mother and her family (*see* Chapter 13). The midwife responsible for the case should be involved in this process.

Professional issues

The midwife should be offered an opportunity to reflect on and discuss the case, in particular the management of the third stage of labour. This may be undertaken with the involvement of the supervisor of midwives.

It is important that documentation accurately reflects the course of events and treatment. As with all obstetric emergencies, if notes are written retrospectively it is necessary to record this fact when documenting the date and times of the events.

References

1 Hofmeyr G, Say L, Gulmezoglu A. (2005) WHO systematic review of maternal mortality and morbidity: the prevalence of uterine rupture. *BJOG.* **112**(9): 1221–8.
2 Porreco R, Clarke S, Belfort M, Diddy G, Meyers J. (2009) The changing specter of uterine rupture. *Am J Obstet Gynecol.* **200**(3): 269–70.
3 Smith G. (2006) Delivery after previous caesarean section. In: James D, Weiner C, Steer P, Gonik B. *High Risk Pregnancy: management options.* 3rd ed. Philadelphia: Saunders.
4 Walsh C, Baxi L. (2007) Rupture of the primigravid uterus: a review of the literature. *Obstet Gynecol Surv.* **62**(5): 327–34.
5 Rogers M, Chang A. (2006) Postpartum hemorrhage and other problems of the third stage. In: James D, Weiner C, Steer P, Gonik B. *High Risk Pregnancy: management options.* 3rd ed. Philadelphia: Saunders.
6 Ofir K, Sheiner E, Lewy A, Katz M, Mazor M. (2004) Uterine rupture: difference between a scarred and an unscarred uterus. *Am J Obstet Gynecol.* **191**(2): 425–9.
7 Kwee A, Bots M, Visser G, *et al.* (2006) Obstetric management and outcome of pregnancy in women with a history of CS in the Netherlands. *Eur J Obstet Gynecol Reprod Biol.* **128**: 257–61.

8   Dow M, Wax J, Pinette M, Blackstone J, Cartin A. (2009) Third-trimester uterine rupture without previous cesarean: a case series and review of the literature. *Am J Perinatol.* **26**(10): 739–44.

9   Gielchinsky Y, Rojansky N, Fasouliotis S, Ezra Y. (2002) Placenta accrete – summary of 10 years: a survey of 310 cases. *Placenta.* **23**: 210–14.

10 Ofir K, Sheiner E, Levy A, Karz M, Mazor M. (2003) Uterine rupture: risk factors and pregnancy outcomes. *Am J Obstet Gynecol.* **189**: 1042–6.

11 Shipp T, Zelop C, Cohen A, Repke J, Lieberman E. (2003) Postcesarean delivery fever and uterine rupture in a subsequent trial of labor. *Obstet Gynecol.* **101**: 136–9.

12 Baskett T. (2004) *Essential Management of Obstetric Emergencies.* 4th ed. Bristol: Clinical Press.

13 Royal College of Obstetricians and Gynaecologists (RCOG). (2007) *Birth after Previous Caesarean Birth. Green-top Guideline No. 45.* London: RCOG.

14 National Institute of Clinical Excellence (NICE). (2004) *Caesarean Section: clinical guideline 13.* London: NICE.

15 Shipp T, Zelop C, Lieberman E. (2008) Assessment of the rate of uterine rupture at the first prenatal visit: a preliminary evaluation. *J Matern Fetal Neonatal Med.* **21**(2): 129–33.

16 Stamilio D, DeFranco E, Pare E, *et al.* (2007) Short interpregnancy interval. Risk of uterine rupture and complications of vaginal birth after cesarean delivery. *Obstet Gynecol.* **110**(5): 1075–82.

17 Bujold E, Mehta SH, Bujold C, *et al.* (2002) Interdelivery interval and uterine rupture. *Am J Obstet Gynecol.* **187**(5): 1199–1202.

18 Algert C, Morris J, Simpson J, *et al.* (2008) Labor before a primary cesarean delivery: reduced risk of uterine rupture in a subsequent trial of labor for vaginal birth after cesarean. *Obstet Gynecol.* **112**(5): 1061–6.

19 Zelop D, Shipp T, Repke J, *et al.* (2000) Effect of previous vaginal delivery on the risk of uterine rupture during a subsequent trial of labor. *Am J Obstet Gynecol.* **183**: 1184–6.

20 Sciscione A, Landon M, Leveno K, *et al.* (2008) Previous preterm cesarean delivery and risk of subsequent uterine rupture. *Obstet Gynecol.* **111**(3): 648–53.

21 Fleisch M, Lux J, Schoppe M, *et al.* (2008) Placenta percreta leading to spontaneous complete uterine rupture in the second trimester. Example of a fatal complication of abnormal placentation following uterine scarring. *Gynecol Obstet Invest.* **65**(2): 80–3.

22 Vaknin A, Maymon R, Mendlovic S, *et al.* (2008) Clinical, sonographic, and epidemiologic features of second- and early third-trimester spontaneous antepartum uterine rupture: a cohort study. *Prenat Diagn.* **28**(6): 478–84.

23 Kaczmarczyk M, Sparen P, Terry P, Cnattingius S. (2007) Risk factors for uterine rupture and neonatal consequences of uterine rupture: a population-based study of successive pregnancy in Sweden. *BJOG.* **114**: 1208–14.

24 Harper L, Macones G. (2008) Predicting success and reducing the risks when attempting vaginal birth after cesarean. *Obstet Gynecol Surv.* **63**(8): 538–45.

25 Cahill A, Waterman B, Stamilio D, *et al.* (2008) Higher maximum doses of oxytocin are associated with an unacceptably high risk for uterine rupture in patients attempting vaginal birth after cesarean delivery. *Am J Obstet Gynecol.* **199**(1): 32.e1–e5.

26 Oladipo A, Syed A. (2008) The views of obstetricians in the south-west of England on the use of prostaglandins and syntocinon in VBAC. *J Obstet Gynaecol.* **28**(2): 177–82.

27 El Kady D, Gilbert W, Xing G, Smith L. (2005) Maternal and neonatal outcomes of assaults during pregnancy. *Obstet Gynecol.* **105**: 357–63.

28 Guise J, McDonagh M, Osterweil P, Nygren P, Chan B, Helfand M. (2004) Systematic review of the incidence and consequences of uterine rupture in women with previous caesarean section. *BMJ.* **329**: 19–25.

29 Matsuo K, Scanlon J, Atlas R, *et al.* (2008) Staircase sign: a newly described uterine contraction pattern seen in rupture

of unscarred gravid uterus. *J Obstet Gynaecol Res.* **34**(1): 100–4.

30 Bujold E, Jastrow N, Simoneau J, *et al.* (2009) Prediction of complete uterine rupture by sonographic evaluation of the lower uterine segment. *Am J Obstet Gynecol.* **201**(3): 320e1–e6.

31 Cheung V. (2008) Sonographic measurement of the lower uterine segment thickness: is it truly predictive of uterine rupture? *J Obstet Gynaecol Can.* **30**(2): 148–51.

32 Kapoor D, Sanjeev D, Alfirevic Z. (2003) Management of unscarred ruptured uterus. *J Perinat Med.* **31**: 337–9.

33 Wykes C. (2007) Uterine inversion. In: Johanson R, Cox C, Grady K, Howell C, editors. *Managing Obstetric Emergencies and Trauma (MOET).* London: RCOG Press.

34 Benedetti T. (2001) Obstetric haemorrhage. In: Gabbe SG, Niebyl JR, Simpson JL, editors. *Obstetrics: normal and problem pregnancies.* 4th ed. New York: Churchill Livingstone.

35 Bhalla R, Wuntakal R, Odejinmi F, Khan R. (2009) Review: acute inversion of the uterus. *Obstet Gynaecol.* **11**: 13–18.

36 Arulkumaran S. (2006) *Emergencies in Obstetrics and Gynaecology.* Oxford: Oxford University Press.

37 Baskett T. (2002) Acute uterine inversion: a review of 40 cases. *J Obstet Gynaecol Can.* **24**: 953–6.

38 Achanna S, Mohamed Z, Krishnan M. (2006) Puerperal uterine inversion: a report of four cases. *J Obstet Gynaecol Res.* **32**(3): 341–5.

39 Kean LH. (2000) Other problems of the third stage. In: Kean LH, Baker PN, Edelstone DI, editors. *Best Practice in Labour Ward Management.* 1st ed. Edinburgh: WB Saunders.

40 Lui D, Rodeck C. (2003) Emergencies in the immediate puerperium. In: Liu D, editor. *Labour Ward Manual.* 3rd ed. Edinburgh: Churchill Livingstone.

41 Hostetler D, Bosworth M. (2000) Uterine inversion: a life-threatening obstetric emergency. *J Am Board Fam Pract.* **13**: 120–3.

42 Ogueh O, Ayida G. (1997) Acute uterine inversion: a new technique of hydrostatic replacement. *BJOG.* **104**: 951–2.

CHAPTER 9

Shoulder dystocia

Caroline Squire

... sometimes the head is so small, and the shoulders so large, that without a very great difficulty they cannot pass, which makes the child remain often in the passage after the head is born. ... When the chirurgeon [surgeon] meets with this case, he must speedily deliver the child out of the prison, for a small delay may there strangle the child.[1] (1697)

Clearly, shoulder dystocia as an obstetric emergency has always existed and it is essential that midwives are fully up to date in their knowledge of what to do when it occurs. Optimal maternal and fetal outcomes are possible if the care providers understand the nature of the problem and the mechanisms involved, have a well-defined management plan and are able to function without undue haste or the use of excessive physical force.[2]

Definition

There are several definitions of shoulder dystocia to be found in the literature and it may be that practitioners use the term in a general sense to describe a range of difficulties encountered with the delivery of the shoulders[3] (*see* Figure 9.1). This lack of consensus has led to variations in the reported incidence of shoulder dystocia and a possible under-reporting of the condition.[4] Furthermore, this lack of consensus has also prevented a true evaluation of the effectiveness of different manoeuvres used in the management of the condition.[5]

Shoulder dystocia is a bony problem which occurs when the anterior or, less commonly, the posterior and, rarely, both fetal shoulders impact on the maternal symphysis pubis and/or the sacral promontory. Currently, shoulder dystocia is defined by the Royal College of Obstetricians and Gynaecologists[6] as 'a delivery that requires additional obstetric manoeuvres to release the shoulders after gentle traction has failed'. Mahran *et al.*[7] feel that failure to use the clinical diagnostic criteria set down by the RCOG has led to over-diagnosis of shoulder dystocia. However, the RCOG[6] definition has been criticised by Melendez *et al.*[8] who feel it to be imprecise and subject to clinician bias.

They consider that the term 'gentle' may be translated differently by different clinicians and this may influence diagnosis. Gibb,[4] however, describes three degrees of shoulder dystocia in order of severity as follows:

- a tight squeeze of a big baby with the normal mechanism of rotation present
- unilateral dystocia where the posterior shoulder has entered the pelvis but the anterior is stuck above the symphysis pubis
- bilateral dystocia where both shoulders are arrested above the pelvic brim.

With the second two types, downward traction will only further impact the shoulders.[9]

Incidence

The incidence of shoulder dystocia is difficult to calculate given the problems in defining it and that the broader the definition, the higher the recorded incidence. However, a range between 0.2% to 3% of all vaginal births has been reported, with an increase in risk as the birth weight increases.[2] In an overview of shoulder dystocia, Baxley and Gobbo[9] report that the incidence of shoulder dystocia increases to 5%–9% among fetuses weighing 4–4.5 kg born to mothers without diabetes. However, Baskett *et al.*[10] conclude that shoulder dystocia is not a predictable birth event since the majority of cases of shoulder dystocia in their study occurred in the absence of increasing birth weight and operative vaginal delivery. Olugbile and Mascarenhas[11] reviewed shoulder dystocia

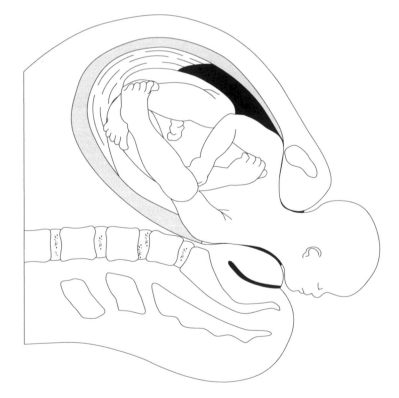

FIGURE 9.1 Shoulder dystocia

at the Birmingham Women's Hospital and the rate of incidence they reported was 0.53%.

Prediction and risk factors

Many authors agree that shoulder dystocia often occurs unexpectedly and the first hint of an impending problem may be slow extension of the fetal head. The chin will remain tight against the mother's perineum and the head may look as though it is trying to return into the vagina ('turtle sign'). Possible risk factors during the preconception period have been identified by O'Leary[12] (*see* Box 9.1).

> **BOX 9.1** Preconception risk factors for shoulder dystocia
> - Macrosomic maternal birth weight
> - Prior birth with shoulder dystocia
> - Prior macrosomic infant
> - Glucose excess states (pre-existing diabetes or obesity)
> - Multiparity
> - Prior gestational diabetes
> - Advanced maternal age.

Currently, there is evidence surrounding links between the rise in maternal obesity and macrosomic fetuses.[13] It may follow that a rise in preconception and antenatal maternal obesity will see a significant rise in incidence of shoulder dystocia.

Cohen *et al.*[14] found that in their study of diabetic patients there was a direct correlation between the level of fetal truncal asymmetry measured sonographically and the incidence and severity of shoulder dystocia. However, Lewis *et al.*[15] found that in their study of data from 1622 women the factors in both the control group and the group of women who experienced shoulder dystocia during their births were not significantly different and included obesity, multiparity, a history of diabetes, short maternal stature, postmaturity and advanced maternal age. Similarly, Blickstein *et al.*[16] found that shoulder dystocia could not be attributed to any particular difference between the current and previous heaviest birth weight. Even in macrosomic infants, they found that shoulder dystocia and brachial plexus injury are unpredictable, although Athukorala *et al.*[17] have found fetal macrosomia to be the strongest independent risk factor for shoulder dystocia in women with gestational diabetes mellitus. In France, Verspyck *et al.*[18] attempted to relate maternal and infant characteristics to the shoulder width of the newborn and to evaluate the predictive value of the shoulder width measurement in cases of shoulder dystocia. They found that although the newborn shoulder width measurement correlated strongly with birth weight, it remained a poor predictor for shoulder dystocia. Gherman *et al.*[2] have also concluded that, although the risk of shoulder dystocia appears to rise with increasing birth weights, 40%–60% of births complicated by shoulder dystocia occur in infants weighing less than 4 kg and 70%–90% of macrosomic infants deliver normally without any pathology.

Ouzounian and Gherman[19] and Baxley and Gobbo[9] have identified the following antenatal risk factors for shoulder dystocia (*see* Box 9.2) and intrapartum risk factors (*see* Box 9.3).

It may be that a combination of risk factors multiply the likelihood of shoulder dystocia and can be predictive in individual cases but identification remains easier with the benefit of hindsight.[9]

> **BOX 9.2** Antenatal risk factors for shoulder dystocia
>
> *Maternal*
> - Abnormal pelvic anatomy
> - Gestational diabetes
> - Post-dates pregnancy
> - Previous shoulder dystocia
> - Short stature
> - Obesity.
>
> *Fetal*
> - Suspected macrosomia.

> **BOX 9.3** Intrapartum risk factors
> - Assisted vaginal delivery (forceps or vacuum)
> - Protracted active phase of first-stage of labour
> - Protracted second-stage of labour
> - Labour augmentation.

Potential maternal outcomes

Baxley and Gobbo[9] have also identified potential maternal trauma (*see* Box 9.4).

> **BOX 9.4** Potential maternal trauma during shoulder dystocia
> - Postpartum haemorrhage
> - Rectovaginal fistula
> - Symphyseal separation or diathesis, with or without transient femoral neuropathy
> - Third or fourth-degree tear or episiotomy
> - Uterine rupture.

It has been reported that shoulder dystocia associated with fundal pressure leading to uterine rupture and catastrophic haemorrhage has resulted in maternal death.[20] The use of fundal pressure, therefore, should be avoided absolutely and considered negligent practice. Importantly, it is likely that the mother and her partner may be emotionally traumatised from their experience and may develop post-traumatic stress disorder even if the infant survives in reasonable health.[21] It may be useful for a midwife to visit them at home, if they wish, to listen to their experiences. Clearly, subsequent births may also be terrifying for the woman and partner and in these situations midwives need to be especially insightful and sensitive.

Potential fetal outcomes

Baxley and Gobbo[9] and Nocon[22] have identified the following potential fetal outcomes (*see* Box 9.5).

> **BOX 9.5** Potential fetal outcomes
> - Brachial plexus injury
> - Phrenic nerve injury
> - Fractures of the clavicle and/or humerus
> - Neonatal asphyxia with, or without permanent neurological damage
> - Fetal death.

Clavicular fractures are among the most common injuries associated with shoulder dystocia, and they also frequently occur in infants weighing less than 4000 g.[22] In terms of neurological damage, Erb's palsy is the result of trauma to the fifth and sixth cervical nerves and manifests with absent biceps and Moro reflex on the affected side. Clinically, there is internal rotation and adduction of the shoulder, an unequal Moro reflex, extension and pronation of the elbow and weak wrist extension or the 'waiter's tip' position.[23] Klumpke's palsy concerns the lower trunk lesion at the eighth cervical and first thoracic vertebrae, generally affecting the intrinsic muscles of the hand, leading to a claw hand that cannot be closed to make a fist. Horner's syndrome may be present on the affected side due to the involvement of the sympathetic fibres that cross the first thoracic vertebra.[24] Rarely, a severe injury will involve the entire plexus and cause complete paralysis of the arm. Another rare injury concerns the fourth cervical root, which involves trauma to the phrenic nerve and would present with features of respiratory distress with paralysed hemidiaphragm.[22]

The highest risk of fractures and neurological damage occurs when traction and fundal pressure are used together to expedite delivery.[25,26] Midwives need to know that fundal pressure must not be used to relieve shoulder dystocia and experts will testify it is a substandard practice in a court of law.[27] McRoberts' manoeuvre, delivery of the posterior arm and corkscrew manoeuvres are associated with the least trauma for both the mother and the infant.[20,28] However, it has been postulated that brachial plexus injury may occur regardless of the procedure used to disimpact the shoulder.[29,30] Gherman *et al.*[31] suggests that brachial plexus palsy and bone fracture may arise as a result of the labour process itself or as an intrauterine event. Brachial plexus injury has been seen to occur after uncomplicated vaginal births, in infants in cephalic presentation during caesarean section and from the posterior shoulder lodging on the sacral promontory.[31-35]

Gonik *et al.*,[34] Yeung Leung and Kwok Hung Chung[36] and Sandmire and DeMott[37] suggest that spontaneous endogenous forces may contribute substantially to neonatal brachial plexus injury and it may be that stopping pushing until the anterior shoulder is freed will limit injury. Nocon[22] concurs, stating that before the midwife or obstetrician is even aware that shoulder dystocia will occur, the brachial plexus may be significantly stretched due to gentle downward traction exerted to assist the birth of the anterior shoulder and the expulsive efforts of the mother driving the anterior shoulder forward and upward above the symphysis. Sandmire and DeMott[37] postulate that the distance over which the brachial plexus is stretched is more important than the amount of maternal force required to enable the birth of the baby. They take the view that the variation in the degree of twisting and the degree of extension of the fetal head and neck in relation to the shoulders during the final movements before birth explains the variation in frequency, severity and persistence of injury to the brachial plexus. Gurewitsch *et al.*[38] found in their retrospective study of neonates with brachial plexus palsies that such palsies were rare without the birth complication of shoulder dystocia. They also found that brachial plexus palsies in neonates whose births were not complicated by shoulder dystocia seemed temporary whereas more than 90% of permanent brachial plexus palsies were associated with births complicated by shoulder dystocia.

Hope *et al.*[39] reviewed the notes of 56 cases of deaths from shoulder dystocia reported to the Confidential Enquiry into Stillbirths and Deaths in Infancy. They found that maternal obesity and big babies were over-represented in pregnancies complicated by fatal shoulder dystocia.

The median time interval between delivery of the head and the rest of the body was only five minutes. This is a very short time interval and they postulated that the reasons for cerebral injury and death in shoulder dystocia may be different to those for cerebral hypoxia-ischaemia from other causes such as cord prolapse or placental abruption. They also suggested that long labour, probably causing metabolic acidosis, compression of the neck resulting in cerebral venous obstruction, excessive vagal stimulation and bradycardia, or other mechanisms, may combine with reduced arterial oxygen supply to cause clinical deterioration out of proportion to the duration of hypoxia. There was evidence from some post mortems that trauma, as well as hypoxia-ischaemia may have contributed to the adverse outcome. Other mechanisms such as massive vagal stimulation would not be detectable at post mortem.

Importantly, Hope et al.[39] found that the midwife was the lead professional at 65% of these births and middle grade or senior obstetric staff were supervising only 47% of the births by the time the body was delivered. Furthermore, they suggest that the delayed arrival of paediatric staff in many cases was less than beneficial, even if there was no guarantee that earlier paediatric intervention would have altered the outcome. Poor communication between parents and professionals was found in several of these cases and they felt that greater involvement of mothers in antenatal and intrapartum decisions may have helped in some cases.

Avoidance of shoulder dystocia

There are three ways to try to reduce the incidence of shoulder dystocia.[17] The first is to deliver all macrosomic fetuses by caesarean section. Indeed, Gross et al.[40] maintained that elective caesarean delivery may be indicated for infants weighing more than 4500 g. Conway[41] presented an overview of the literature with regard to the vexed question of delivery of the macrosomic infant of a diabetic woman and whether it should be by caesarean section or vaginal birth. In her study she found that the shoulder dystocia rate among macrosomic infants (over 4000 g) born vaginally was significantly higher than among appropriately grown infants, and the rate among diabetic women was higher than among non-diabetics. She came to the following conclusions:

1 Shoulder dystocia and brachial plexus injury risk increase with increasing birth weight in infants of diabetic mothers.

2 Caesarean delivery essentially eliminates the risk of brachial plexus injury.

3 Use of a fetal weight threshold for recommending caesarean delivery, when fetal weight is determined by ultrasonography, can result in a decrease in the occurrence of shoulder dystocia in diabetic women.

4 The benefit of reducing the shoulder dystocia rate in diabetic women (and thereby reducing the rate of permanent brachial plexus injuries) must be weighed carefully against the maternal cost of increased caesarean deliveries with their associated short and long-term morbidities.

5 Fetal overgrowth is best detected ultrasonographically by employing fetal weight formulae in common clinical use.

However, although this would obviate the trauma described above to the mother and fetus the suggestion of elective caesarean section has been criticised because it is difficult to predict macrosomic infants even with the use of ultrasound.[9,42–44] Studies have shown that there is a marked increase in caesarean section for babies with a heavy birth weight predicted before delivery but with no significant difference in the incidence of shoulder dystocia or birth trauma.[45,46] Data collected by Blickstein *et al.*[16] suggest that birth weights of more than 4200 g carry a risk of 1:8–9 for shoulder dystocia and 1:79 for brachial plexus injury while Zafeiriou and Psychogiou[46] and Raio *et al.*[47] found that there was a higher incidence of brachial plexus injury in fetuses with a birth weight of more than 4500 g. To add to the picture, Iffy *et al.*[48] published a retrospective analysis of 316 fetal neurological injuries associated with deliveries complicated by arrest of the shoulders that occurred across the USA. They concluded that current North American and British guidelines that set 5000 g as minimum estimated fetal weight limit for elective caesarean section in non-diabetic women and 4500 g for diabetic pregnant women may expose some macrosomic fetuses to a high risk of permanent neurological damage. The issue of prevention of shoulder dystocia through the use of caesarean section remains cloudy with the particular difficulty of estimating fetal birth weight accurately and, then, translating that knowledge into appropriate practice.

The second way to try to reduce the incidence of shoulder dystocia is to avoid macrosomia by inducing suspected cases. However, it seems clear that induction of labour and ripening of a relatively unripe cervix contributes to an excessive caesarean delivery rate with its concomitant hazards. There is also a risk of iatrogenic prematurity, especially in the early delivery of the diabetic mother. In addition there is the problem of accurate estimation of fetal weight by ultrasound given its wide margin of error at term as discussed before.

In a Cochrane systematic review, Irion and Boulvain[49] evaluated a policy of labour induction for suspected fetal macrosomia on the risk of perinatal trauma or asphyxia. They found that there is currently no evidence that a systematic policy of labour induction for suspected fetal macrosomia in non-diabetic women can reduce maternal or neonatal morbidity. However, they only considered three randomised controlled trials with a small sample size to evaluate this intervention and recommended larger randomised controlled trials with enough power to detect an effect of induction of labour as a policy.

However, it may be that the obstetrician should make a clinical evaluation and opt for induction if the cervix is ripe and the woman is at term.[22]

The third way to attempt to reduce the incidence of shoulder dystocia is to identify any antenatal indicators for the complication (*see* Boxes 9.1 and 9.2) with a view to influencing decisions surrounding timing and method of birth. This may raise questions, for example, such as whether babies of diabetic mothers be delivered by caesarean section before 40 weeks' gestation. Although a policy of elective caesarean delivery may be more justifiable in this population, it is still controversial. Nesbitt *et al.*[43] found that the risk of shoulder dystocia for unassisted and assisted births to diabetic mothers increased as the birth weight increased. Hankins *et al.*[50] published a review of the literature for the previous 10 years in the USA to consider caesarean section on request at 39 weeks' gestation. They looked at the impact on various areas of neonatal trauma to include the sequelae of shoulder dystocia in terms of permanent brachial plexus injury. They calculated that the range for permanent brachial plexus injury that could be avoided with caesarean section on request would appear to vary between 1:5000 and 1:10 000 vaginal births and, therefore, cannot be recommended. However, Draycott *et al.*[51] report that in a subgroup of women with diabetes with suspected fetal macrosomia or where the estimated fetal weight is over 5000 g in women without diabetes, elective caesarean section can be recommended because of the higher incidence of shoulder dystocia and brachial plexus injury in this subgroup. Boulvain, Stan and Irion[52] performed a systematic review for the Cochrane Collaboration to consider elective delivery in diabetic pregnant women. They found a paucity of quality research and only managed to review one randomised controlled trial which compared induction of labour with expectant management in insulin-requiring diabetic pregnant women at term. This trial found that the risk of macrosomia, defined as birth weight above 4000 g, was reduced in the active induction group. No incidences of mild shoulder dystocia were reported in the induction group as opposed to three cases in the expectant management group. Clearly, more research is required here.

Management at birth
Diagnosis
Timely recognition and accurate management of shoulder dystocia are imperative in preventing birth trauma to the mother

and fetus (*see* Box 9.3 for risk factors). The fetal head is born, typically after a long period of bearing down by the exhausted mother, and retracts or recoils against the maternal perineum and then fails to restitute in line with the shoulders. The retraction of the fetal head is known as the 'turtle sign'.[53] Even if external rotation is accomplished, lateral traction of normal force is ineffective in delivering the anterior shoulder beneath the symphysis. Forceful lateral traction should be avoided as this is likely to cause greater impaction of the shoulders against the pelvic inlet and the mother should be asked not to bear down for the same reason and, also, to prevent exacerbation of prior stretching of brachial plexus.[51]

Help should be summoned immediately by pulling the emergency buzzer and asking for the coordinating midwife, another midwife, senior obstetrician, paediatrician and the anaesthetist. Someone should be asked to take over the writing of the notes and another to set up the resuscitaire, put the heater on, set the timer and warm the towels for the baby. The notes should contain the following information and be signed clearly and dated:

1 The time of the delivery of the head
2 The time assistance was called, the staff that were called
3 The time the staff in attendance arrived
4 The manoeuvres performed, the timing and the sequence
5 The traction applied
6 The condition of the baby.

If shoulder dystocia occurs at a home birth, the ambulance should be called urgently and transfer to hospital should be as swift as possible in order to gain access to neonatal resuscitation facilities. The maternity unit should be informed of what is happening prior to arrival. A situation such as this serves to emphasise the importance of having two midwives present at home births so that one can make the necessary telephone calls to summon assistance, keep times of key events such as the birth of the fetal head and maintain contemporaneous records. Both can help the other in terms of clinical decision making, neonatal resuscitation and giving emotional support to the mother and family and each other.

Manoeuvres to expedite delivery

The various manoeuvres are described below. It is important to realise, however, that no single manoeuvre has been proven to be superior to any other in disimpacting the shoulder and none is entirely free from potential injury to the fetus or mother.[22] Nocon[22] found that regardless of the manoeuvre used, about 15%–20% of infants suffer some injury, albeit transitory. He feels that no protocol should serve as a substitute for clinical judgement because there is no rationale for choosing one technique over another.

Although shoulder dystocia is rare it creates an urgent situation, so there should be regular multidisciplinary review and reflection on manoeuvres. A mnemonic designed to help midwives and other clinicians involved with births complicated by shoulder dystocia is described in Box 9.6. It is important to understand that the mnemonic serves to illustrate a variety of manoeuvres that can be used and, though it is better to consider external manoeuvres first, the order of these actions may be different from the order in Box 9.6. It is up to the clinician at the time who is aware of the particular circumstances to decide which seem the best actions to do and in which order.

BOX 9.6 Drill for shoulder dystocia (adapted from the Advanced Life Support in Obstetrics course[54])

H Help! Call for help; activate protocol.

E Evaluate for episiotomy: enables better access to the fetus and for internal manoeuvres.

L Legs: McRoberts' manoeuvre (30–60 seconds).

P Pressure: external suprapubic (30–60 seconds).

E Enter the vagina: Woods' screw; Rubin's (30–60 seconds).

R Remove the posterior arm.

R Roll over onto all fours.

Disimpaction manoeuvres
The McRoberts' manoeuvre

This manoeuvre involves removing pillows from the mother's back, lying her flat and bringing her to the end of the bed or removing the end of the bed to make vaginal access easier. With one assistant on either side, her legs are hyperflexed against her abdomen as far as is possible (*see* Figure 9.2). It has been associated with lower levels of maternal and fetal morbidity.[28] When used alone, McRoberts' manoeuvre has alleviated approximately 40% of all shoulder dystocia cases and this rises to 54% when it is combined with suprapubic pressure. Furthermore, its use can reduce fetal shoulder extraction force and brachial plexus stretching which may help reduce the incidence of

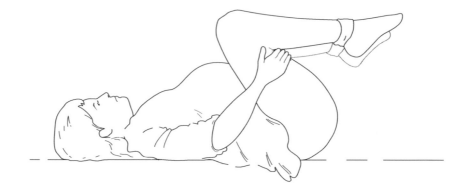

FIGURE 9.2 McRoberts' manoeuvre

palsy due to brachial plexus damage.[55] Gherman *et al.*[56] analysed the McRoberts' manoeuvre by X-ray pelvimetry and found that it does not change the actual dimension of the maternal pelvis, but that it does straighten the sacrum relative to the lumbar spine and may enable the symphysis pubis to rotate superiorly and slide over the fetal shoulder.

It also reduces the angle of inclination. Smeltzer[57] considers that the McRoberts' manoeuvre elevates the anterior fetal shoulder and flexes the fetal spine. The action of lifting and flexion pushes the posterior shoulder over the sacrum and through the pelvic inlet and straightens the maternal spine. Also, the superior rotation of the symphysis pubis will bring the plane of the pelvic inlet perpendicular to the maximum maternal expulsive force. It is thought that a limitation of McRoberts' manoeuvre is that the fetal shoulders are maintained in the smaller anteroposterior diameter of the pelvis.[58]

The McRoberts' manoeuvre is recommended as the initial technique in the management of shoulder dystocia because it does not involve manipulation of the fetus and would seem to be relatively safe. However, Gherman *et al.*[59] published a case study in which it seemed that symphysis separation and transient femoral neuropathy were associated with this manoeuvre. They postulate that an overly exaggerated lithotomy position and thigh abduction stretches the articular surfaces of the symphysis pubis and that increased pressure is placed on the femoral nerve by the overlying inguinal ligament. Heath and Gherman[60] reported a case of symphysis separation and sacro-iliac dislocation resulting from excessive or prolonged maternal hip flexion.

If there is no movement of the fetal shoulders, the next manoeuvre can be performed.

Suprapubic pressure

Suprapubic pressure is another non-invasive disimpaction manoeuvre and should be considered as a second step because its use may result in clavicular fractures. Before suprapubic pressure is attempted, the maternal bladder should be empty to avoid bladder trauma and impediment to shoulder rotation. The method advocated is to apply gentle pressure with the palm or the heel of the hand against the fetal back, directing the pressure towards the fetal midline (*see* Figure 9.3). This can be performed also using a compression/ relaxation cycle analogous to cardiopulmonary resuscitation.⁹ This will adduct the shoulders and may decrease the bisacromial diameter, allowing the shoulder to rotate off the pubic bone and into the wider oblique diameter of the pelvic inlet. It may also shift the anterior shoulder into the wider oblique diameter of the pelvic brim. Usually, this procedure is used in conjunction with other manoeuvres, commonly the McRoberts' manoeuvre.

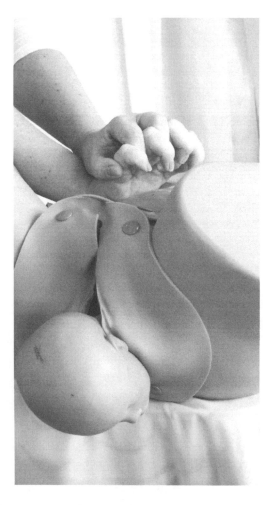

FIGURE 9.3 Suprapubic pressure

Clearly, it is important to know the position of the fetus beforehand otherwise the bisacromial diameter will increase and cause the situation to become even more serious. As mentioned above, it is possible to use the McRoberts' manoeuvre and suprapubic pressure at the same time, in which case the incidence of resolution rises to 54%.⁵⁶

All-fours or Gaskin manoeuvre

If the McRobert's manoeuvre is not the most appropriate initial response to suspected shoulder dystocia, women and midwives may find the all-fours position useful. The actual movement of the woman turning onto her hands and knees may help dislodge the shoulder, particularly if it is the posterior shoulder that is impacted behind the sacral promontory, although the anterior shoulder could remain wedged against the symphysis pubis. However, the midwife loses eye contact with the mother, which may make communication at this crucial time more difficult. Bruner *et al.*⁶¹ felt that the all-fours manoeuvre appeared to be a rapid, safe and effective technique for reducing shoulder dystocia in labouring women and reported an 83% success rate in one case series. They were enthusiastic in their appraisal of the manoeuvre and make it clear that the all-fours position does not preclude the performance of the other manoeuvres, such as the McRoberts' manoeuvre, suprapubic pressure, shoulder rotation, delivery of the posterior arm and even cephalic replacement. Kovavisarach⁶² also presents a positive opinion on this manoeuvre by publishing a case study of a woman who had shoulder dystocia. All other manoeuvres had been exhausted but the baby was delivered seemingly without much problem following the mother turning onto the all-fours position.

Rotation manoeuvres and manoeuvres involving manipulation of the fetus

If the McRoberts' manoeuvre and suprapubic pressure have not been successful, the next line of action is the internal rotational manoeuvres and delivery of the posterior arm. The aims of internal rotation are:

1 To move the fetal shoulders (bisacromial diameter) out of the narrowest diameter (anteroposterior) of the mother's pelvis and into a wider pelvic diameter (oblique – more likely – or transverse).
2 To reduce fetal bisacromial diameter.

Vaginal access should always be gained posteriorly via the sacral hollow. There is more room here to make access easier for the clinician and, importantly, less painful for the mother without an epidural.

Woods' screw rotational manoeuvre

This involves the midwife placing two fingers into the vagina against the anterior chest wall opposite the posterior shoulder and pushing the posterior shoulder backwards through a 180-degree arc (*see* Figure 9.4). As the posterior shoulder rotates, it may deliver or it may free the anterior shoulder for delivery. However, this manoeuvre may result in the abduction of the shoulders, which increases the bisacromial diameter and complicates the problem. For this reason, suprapubic pressure may be applied concurrently to keep the anterior shoulder adducted.[63]

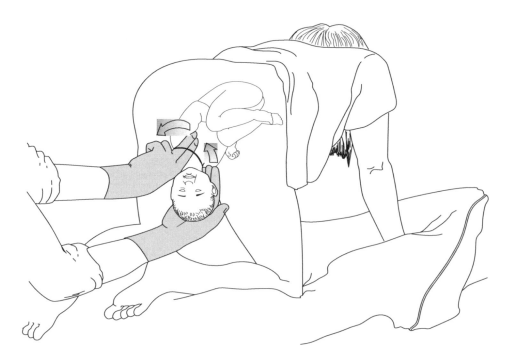

FIGURE 9.4 Woods' screw rotational manoeuvre

The Rubin manoeuvre

The aim of this manoeuvre is to reduce the bisacromial diameter by adducting the fetal shoulders and it involves the midwife inserting two fingers into the mother's vagina onto the posterior shoulder of the fetus (*see* Figure 9.5). The posterior shoulder may then be displaced by the application of pressure in the direction of the fetal chest.[63] This manoeuvre may be more effective than the Woods' screw manoeuvre because it keeps the shoulders in a forward position or adducted, reducing the bisacromial diameter. Suprapubic pressure may also be applied here so that the anterior shoulder is rocked by pushing from side to side on the mother's abdomen. This may free the anterior shoulder and give the posterior shoulder room to turn.[64]

A variation of the Rubin manoeuvre has also been described as the **reverse** Woods' screw manoeuvre. Several fingers are placed into the vagina via the sacral hollow and then gently moved up against the surface of the scapula of the anterior shoulder which is then rotated forward through a 180-degree arc (*see* Figure 9.6). The application of digital pressure onto the anterior shoulder should only be performed if pressure onto the posterior shoulder has not been successful because there is so little room between the scapula and the pubic bone and the manoeuvre would cause intolerable pain to the mother who does not have an epidural *in situ*. If the posterior shoulder is more accessible, it may be rotated anteriorly. Whichever shoulder is manoeuvred, the principle is the same so that the shoulders are adducted in order to reduce the bisacromial diameter and free the wedged shoulder.

Whichever rotational manoeuvre is

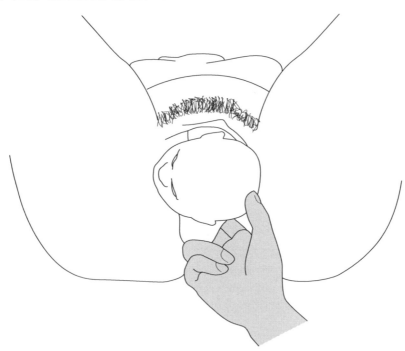

FIGURE 9.5 Rubin manoeuvre

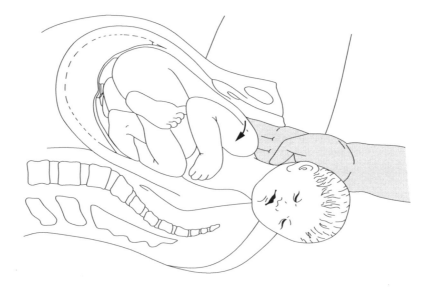

FIGURE 9.6 Reverse Woods' screw manoeuvre

used from within the pelvis, a second clinician can perform suprapubic pressure to assist rotation. Communication needs to be clear between each other so that both work together to ensure that they are pushing in the same direction and not against each other.

Recent alternative developments in rotational manoeuvres: entering the vagina

Draycott *et al.*[51] have published a manual entitled *Practical Obstetric Multiprofessional Training* – PROMPT – which has much to commend it. The key development therein is that they feel that attempting to gain access to the vagina anteriorly is very difficult because there is hardly any room between the subpubic arch and the anterior shoulder trapped underneath the symphysis pubis and advocate that this should be considered incorrect practice. They suggest that the

midwife scrunches up (makes a cone shape of) her hand as if trying to put on a tight bracelet so that the whole hand can be used to enter the vagina via the posterior sacral hollow to perform the internal rotational manoeuvres considered previously (*see* Figure 9.7). This will mean that the midwife will have more power of leverage to compensate for the use of only the one hand and will have the additional advantage that the shoulders may be adducted.

Draycott *et al.*[51] advocate, therefore, that the clinician attempts rotation by:
1 Applying pressure from the scrunched hand onto the posterior aspect of the posterior shoulder to enable rotation of the shoulders to the wider oblique diameter and facilitation of birth. If delivery does not occur then:
2 Continue pressure and, by swapping hands, rotate the shoulders 180 degrees. This should substitute the anterior shoulder for the posterior shoulder and,

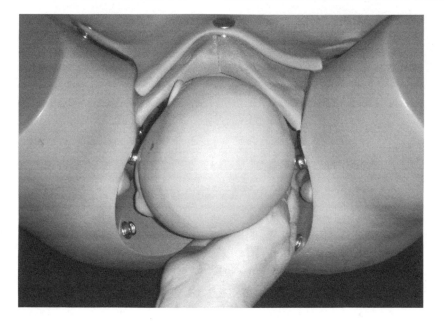

FIGURE 9.7 Scrunched/coned hand

hopefully, delivery should follow. If delivery does not occur then:

3 Try to rotate the shoulders in the opposite direction by applying pressure using a scrunched hand onto the anterior aspect of the fetal posterior shoulder. If delivery does not occur then:

4 Apply pressure onto the posterior aspect of the anterior fetal shoulder by entering via the sacral hollow and following the fetal back as far as the scapula. This is a manoeuvre that Draycott *et al.*[51] feel should not be attempted unless necessary due to the difficulty and discomfort that may be inflicted onto the woman (see above); attempt to adduct and rotate the shoulders into the wider oblique diameter.

Delivery of the posterior arm

Delivery of the posterior arm is attempted when rotational manoeuvres fail to relieve the impaction of the fetus that is tightly wedged into the pelvic brim or when the midwife or clinician feels that it is possible. This will reduce the diameter of the fetal shoulders by the width of the arm or 20% of the shoulder diameter[65] and may well resolve the shoulder dystocia.[66] The midwife places two fingers into the vagina via the sacral hollow and follows the humerus from the posterior shoulder to the elbow (*see* Figure 9.8). Pressure into the antecubital fossa will help the forearm to flex so that it can be swept over the chest. Delivery of the arm may facilitate rotation of the fetus through a 180-degree arc, bringing the posterior shoulder under the symphysis pubis and allowing the rest of the birth to be completed normally.[64] Trauma, such as fracture of the humerus or clavicle, may occur if the arm is tightly wedged, but this may be considered comparatively unimportant at this stage.[9]

The point at which the clinician decides

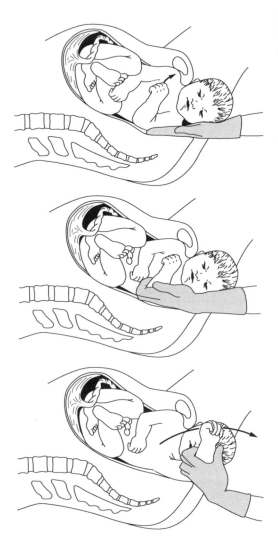

FIGURE 9.8 Delivery of the posterior arm

to attempt delivery of the posterior arm varies according to the judgement of the clinician at the time. This illustrates that the HELPERR mnemonic serves to present a repertoire of different actions in some sort of order that can be executed in challenging situations, but it is not meant to be used literally on every occasion. In the RCOG Guideline No. 42[6] the suggestion is to consider attempting to deliver the posterior arm earlier in

the management of this emergency (*see* Figure 9.9). It depends on the view of the clinician at the time.

Surgical procedures
Episiotomy
An episiotomy is usually performed in order to give extra space at the introitus for the clinician to attempt any direct manoeuvres or manipulation of the fetus. It may be that damage to the perineum is lessened in the long term, although Gurewitsch *et al.*[68] postulate that in severe shoulder dystocia, if fetal manipulation can be performed without episiotomy, severe perineal trauma can be averted without incurring greater risk of brachial plexus palsy.

Symphysiotomy
This is the surgical division of the fibro-cartilage junction of the symphysis pubis to enlarge the bony pelvis and has been practised for many years in areas of the world where caesarean section is difficult to perform. The procedure is not widely practised in the UK or the USA, possibly due to operator inexperience and maternal morbidity.[69,70] Three case studies were published concerning the use of this procedure. In all cases the infants died, although it should be remembered that all the standard manoeuvres including cephalic replacement had already been performed to no avail and symphysiotomy was performed *in extremis*. Maternal morbidity, including urinary incontinence, was significant but responded to treatment,[69] and Chalidis *et al.*[71] describe the management and reconstruction of pelvic instability after emergency symphysiotomy with the use of plates to fix and hold the symphysis pubis in place.

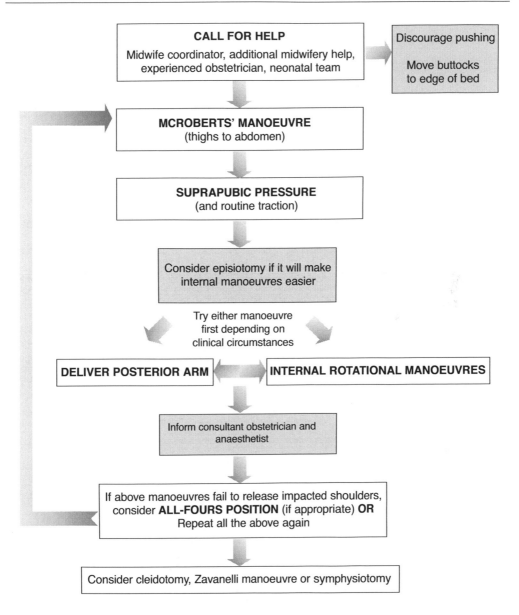

CALL FOR HELP

Midwife coordinator, additional midwifery help, experienced obstetrician, neonatal team

Discourage pushing

Move buttocks to edge of bed

MCROBERTS' MANOEUVRE
(thighs to abdomen)

SUPRAPUBIC PRESSURE
(and routine traction)

Consider episiotomy if it will make internal manoeuvres easier

Try either manoeuvre first depending on clinical circumstances

DELIVER POSTERIOR ARM ◄► **INTERNAL ROTATIONAL MANOEUVRES**

Inform consultant obstetrician and anaesthetist

If above manoeuvres fail to release impacted shoulders, consider **ALL-FOURS POSITION** (if appropriate) **OR** Repeat all the above again

Consider cleidotomy, Zavanelli manoeuvre or symphysiotomy

Baby to be reviewed by neonatologist

DOCUMENT ON PRO FORMA AND COMPLETE CLINICAL INCIDENT REPORTING FORM

FIGURE 9.9 Algorithm for the management of shoulder dystocia (reproduced with the permission of the RCOG)

Cephalic replacement: Zavanelli manoeuvre

The Zavanelli manoeuvre involves replacing the fetal head into the pelvis for extraction by caesarean section. The head is rotated to a direct occipitoanterior or occipitoposterior position and flexed. Then pressure is applied to the vertex to push the head upwards.[73,74] Various case studies have been published concerning this manoeuvre but at the present time, although it is thought that it should be on every obstetrician's list, it must remain a low priority until its applicability has been demonstrated more clearly.[73–76] Severe injuries associated with the Zavanelli manoeuvre, though not necessarily as a result, include Erb's palsy, paresis of the lower extremities, seizures, brain damage, delayed motor development, quadriplegia, cerebral palsy and neonatal death. Reported maternal complications have included uterine infection requiring hysterectomy, vaginal 'rupture', laceration of the lower uterine segment and uterine rupture.[64]

Delivery in subsequent pregnancies

Smith[77] studied 51 case notes of women who had experienced previous births complicated by shoulder dystocia. In the subsequent pregnancy, five women underwent elective caesarean birth, including four of the five diabetic mothers. Four women had emergency caesarean sections in labour for fetal hypoxia, placental abruption and failure to progress. Of the 42 women delivering vaginally, five experienced a repeated episode of shoulder dystocia. There were no episodes of fetal death or trauma. This gave a repeat recurrence of 9.8% as compared with the total population incidence of 0.58%.

Overland *et al.*[78] published a retrospective cohort study aiming to estimate the relative and absolute risk of shoulder dystocia in the second birth according to a history of shoulder dystocia and the older child's birth weight. Their study included all women in Norway with two consecutive singleton vaginal births with the fetus in cephalic presentation during the period 1967–2005. They found that

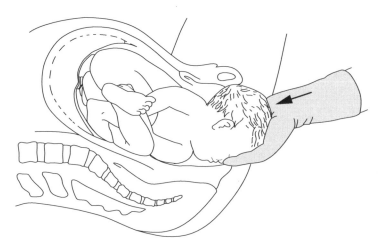

FIGURE 9.10 Zavanelli manoeuvre

in the second delivery, shoulder dystocia occurred in 0.8% of all women. In women with a prior shoulder delivery the recurrence risk was 7.3%. However, they found that most incidences of shoulder dystocia in the second birth were in women without such history – 96.2%. They found that the elder child's birth weight was the most important risk factor for shoulder dystocia in the second birth.

Moore *et al.*[79] performed a population-based case control study to evaluate the incidence of, and risk factors for, recurrence of shoulder dystocia in women attempting subsequent vaginal birth. They found that a birth weight of 3500 g or more, vacuum delivery or severe shoulder dystocia previously were independent risk factors for recurrence of shoulder dystocia. Their finding of a birth weight of 3500 g as a baseline for becoming an independent risk factor for recurrence of shoulder dystocia is surprising and is lower than studies mentioned above.

The best way to manage subsequent births following one complicated with shoulder dystocia remains unclear, but it is important to use what information there is in the literature to form a rational and reasonable management plan for risk modification and for management of a shoulder dystocia event should it recur.[80] Certainly, the wishes of the mother are central, as are the clinical picture and the judgement of health professionals at the time.

Training to improve management of shoulder dystocia

It is now evident that training of midwives and obstetric staff in the management of shoulder dystocia improves outcomes at delivery.[81–84]

Draycott *et al.*[82] compared 15 908 pretraining births with 13 117 births occurring after the introduction of training of the management of shoulder dystocia in their retrospective observational study. Pretraining, they found that none of the recommended manoeuvres for the resolution for shoulder dystocia was used in half or more of the infants that suffered serious morbidity to include brachial plexus damage. After training, at least one of the recommended manoeuvres was utilised in more than 90% of the cases of shoulder dystocia and the risk of neonatal injury decreased significantly from 9.3% to 2.3%.

Heazell and Bhatti[83] found substantial gains in the use of a mnemonic to improve the management of shoulder dystocia. They published research which included a retrospective case notes-based study to describe practice prior to the introduction of a mnemonic and also a prospective study to evaluate the use of a mnemonic in practice and whether this had an effect on fetal morbidity. In the retrospective study, they found that care was given in an unstructured non-evidence-based manner in 35% of incidences and documentation was incomplete in 68% of cases. There was a 5% incidence of injury to the infant. Following the introduction of a mnemonic the use of evidence-based manoeuvres increased to 100%, care was delivered in a structured manner and there were no recorded incidences of injuries to infants.

When introducing training programmes into maternity units for the management of shoulder dystocia, it would seem sensible to repeat these programmes several times a year so that midwives and obstetricians retain skills through repetition. Crofts *et al.*[84] researched skill retention six and 12 months after shoulder dystocia training and found that the large majority of participants retained their newly acquired skills at six and 12 months. They concluded that, overall, training resulted in a sustained improvement in performance and that annual training seemed adequate for those already proficient before training but more frequent rehearsal would be advisable for those initially lacking competency until skill acquisition was achieved. It is likely that their results were so favourable partly because participants would have practised beforehand before they were tested, but that is to be welcomed.

Checklist for midwives

- Enact the HELPERR mnemonic (*see* Box 9.6).
- Remember record keeping.
- Communicate with the mother and her birth partner. Help her/them debrief later if appropriate.
- Practise the manoeuvres.
- Reflect on your experiences with peers and/or Supervisor of Midwives
- Consider risk management issues.

References

1 Chamberlen H. (1697) *The Diseases of Women with Child, and in Child-bed.* 3rd ed. London: Andrew Bell.
2 Gherman RB, Chauhan S, Ouzounian JG, Lerner H, Gonik B, Goodwin TM. (2006) Shoulder dystocia: the unpreventable obstetric emergency with empiric management guidelines. *Am J Obstet Gynecol.* 195(3): 657–72.
3 Mortimore VR, McNabb M. (1998) A six-year retrospective analysis of shoulder dystocia and delivery of the shoulders. *Midwifery.* 14: 162–73.
4 Gibb D. (1995) Clinical focus: shoulder dystocia: the obstetrics. *Clin Focus.* 1: 49–54.
5 Maternal and Child Health Research Consortium. (1995) *Confidential Enquiry into Stillbirth and Deaths in Infancy (Second Annual Report).* London: CESDI.
6 Royal College of Obstetricians and Gynaecologists (RCOG). (2005) *Shoulder Dystocia: Greentop Guideline No. 42.* London: RCOG.
7 Mahran MA, Sayed AT, Imoh-Ita F. (2008) Avoiding over diagnosis of shoulder dystocia. *J Obstet Gynaecol.* 28(2): 173–6.
8 Melendez V, Forson V, Yoong W. (2009) Letter to the editor: Re: Mahran MA, Sayed AT, Imoh-Ita F. (2008) Avoiding over diagnosis of shoulder dystocia. *J Obstet Gynaecol.* 28(2): 173–6.
9 Baxley EG, Gobbo RW. (2004) Shoulder dystocia. *Am Fam Physician.* 69(7): 1707–14.
10 Baskett TF, Allen VM, O'Connell CM, Allen AC. (2007) Fetal trauma in term pregnancy. *Am J Obstet Gynecol.* 197: 499.e1–e7.
11 Olugbile A, Mascarenhas L. (2000) Review of shoulder dystocia at the Birmingham Women's Hospital. *J Obstet Gynaecol.* 20(3): 267–70.
12 O'Leary JA. (1993) Cephalic replacement for shoulder dystocia: present status and future role of the Zavanelli maneuver. *Obstet Gynecol.* 82: 847–50.
13 Ay L, Kruithof CJ, Bakkar R, Steepers EAP, *et al.* (2009) Maternal anthropometrics are associated with fetal size in different periods of pregnancy and at birth. The Generation R Study. *Br J Obstet Gynaecol.* 117(7): 953–63.
14 Cohen BF, Penning S, Ansley D, Porto M, Garite T. (1999) The incidence and severity of shoulder dystocia correlates with a sonographic measurement of asymmetry in patients with diabetes. *Am J Perinatol.* 16(4): 197–201.
15 Lewis DF, Edwards MS, Asrat T, *et al.* (1998) Can shoulder dystocia be predicted? *J Reprod Med.* 43(8): 654–8.
16 Blickstein I, Ben-Arie A, Hagay ZJ. (1998) Antepartum risks of shoulder dystocia and

brachial plexus injury for infants weighing 4200 g or more. *Gynecol Obstet Invest.* **45**: 77–80.

17 Athukorala C, Crowther CA, Willson K. (2007) Women with gestational diabetes mellitus in the ACHOIS trial: risk factors for shoulder dystocia. *Aust N Z J Obstet Gynaecol.* **47**(1): 37–41.

18 Verspyck E, Goffinet F, Hellow MF, *et al.* (1999) Newborn shoulder width: a prospective study of 2222 consecutive measurements. *Br J Obstet Gynaecol.* **106**: 589–92.

19 Ouzounian JG, Gherman RB. (2005) Shoulder dystocia: are historic risk factors reliable predictors? *Am J Obstet Gynecol.* **192**: 1933.

20 Al-Najashi S, Al-Suleiman SA, El-Yahia A, *et al.* (1989) Shoulder dystocia – a clinical study of 56 cases. *Aust N Z J Obstet Gynaecol.* **29**: 129–31.

21 Menage J. (1996) Post traumatic stress disorder following obstetric/ gynaecological procedures. *Br J Midwif.* **4**(10): 532–3.

22 Nocon JJ. (2000) Shoulder dystocia and macrosomia. In: Kean LH, Baker PN, Edelstone DI, editors. *Best Practice in Labour Ward Management.* London: WB Saunders.

23 Ubachs JMH, Slooff ACJ, Peeters LLH. (1995) Obstetric antecedents of surgically treated obstetric brachial plexus injuries. *Br J Obstet Gynaecol.* **102**: 813–17.

24 Swaiman KF, Wright FS. (1982) *The Practice of Pediatric Neurology.* 2nd ed. St Louis: Mosby.

25 Gross SJ, Shime J, Farine D. (1987) Shoulder dystocia: predictors and outcome: a five year review. *Am J Obstet Gynecol.* **56**(2): 334–6.

26 Bahar AM. (1996) Risk factors and fetal outcome in cases of shoulder dystocia compared with normal deliveries of a similar birth weight. *Br J Obstet Gynaecol.* **103**: 868–72.

27 Tolin J. (1992) The attorney's viewpoint. In: O'Leary JA, editor. *Shoulder Dystocia and Birth Injury: prevention and treatment.* New York: McGraw Hill.

28 Gherman RB, Goodwin TM, Souter I, *et al.* (1997) The McRoberts' maneuver for the alleviation of shoulder dystocia: how successful is it? *Am J Obstet Gynecol.* **176**(3): 656–61.

29 Lerner HM, Salamon E. (2008) Permanent brachial plexus injury following vaginal delivery without physician traction or shoulder dystocia Case Report. *Am J Obstet Gynecol.* March: e7–e8.

30 McFarland MB, Langer O, Piper JM, Berkus MD. (1996) Perinatal outcome and the type and number of maneuvers in shoulder dystocia. *Int J Obstet Gynecol.* **55**: 219–24.

31 Gherman RB, Goodwin TM, Ouzounian JG. (1997) Brachial plexus palsy associated with cesarean section: an in utero injury? *Am J Obstet Gynecol.* **177**: 1162–4.

32 Jennett RJ, Tarby TJ, Kreinick CJ. (1992) Brachial plexus palsy: an old problem revisited. *Am J Obstet Gynecol.* **166**: 1673–7.

33 Gherman RB, Ouzounian JG, Miller DA, *et al.* (1998) Spontaneous vaginal delivery: a risk factor for Erb's palsy. *Am J Obstet Gynecol.* **178**: 423–7.

34 Gonik B, Walker A, Grimm M. (2000) Mathematic modelling of forces associated with shoulder dystocia: a comparison of endogenous and exogenous sources. *Am J Obstet Gynecol.* **182**: 689–91.

35 Hankins GDV, Clark SL. (1995) Brachial plexus palsy involving the posterior shoulder at spontaneous vaginal delivery. *Am J Obstet Gynecol.* **12**: 44–5.

36 Yeung Leung T, Kwok Hung Chung T. (2009) Severe chronic morbidity following childbirth. *Best Pract Res Clin Obstet Gynaecol.* doi:10.1016/j. bpobgyn.2009.01.002.

37 Sandmire HF, DeMott RK. (2009) Controversies surrounding the causes of brachial plexus injury. *Int J Gynaecol Obstet.* **104**: 9–13.

38 Gurewitsch ED, Johnson E, Hamzehzadeh S, Allen RH. (2006) Risk factors for brachial plexus injury with and without shoulder dystocia. *Am J Obstet Gynecol.* **194**: 486–92.

39 Hope P, Breslin S, Lamont L, *et al.* (1998) Fatal shoulder dystocia: a review of 56

cases reported to the confidential enquiry into stillbirths and deaths in infancy. *Br J Obstet Gynaecol.* **105**: 1256–61.

40 Gross TL, Sokol RJ, Williams T, *et al.* (1987) Shoulder dystocia: a fetal–physician risk. *Am J Obstet Gynecol.* **156**: 1408–18.

41 Conway DL. (2002) Delivery of the macrosomic infant: cesarean section versus vaginal delivery. *Semin Perinatol.* **26**(3): 225–31.

42 Gherman RB, Joseph G, Ouzounian JG, Murphy Goodwin T. (1998) Obstetric maneuvers for shoulder dystocia and associated fetal morbidity. *Am J Obstet Gynecol.* **178**(6): 1126–30.

43 Nesbitt TS, Gilbert WM, Herrchen B. (1998) Shoulder dystocia and associated risk factors with macrosomic infants born in California. *Am J Obstet Gynecol.* **179**: 476–80.

44 Chauhan SP, Grobman WA, Gherman RA, Chauhan VB, Chang G, Magann EF. (2005) Suspicion and treatment of the macrosomic fetus: a review. *Am J Obstet Gynecol.* **193**: 332–46.

45 Levine AB, Lockwood CJ, Brown B, *et al.* (1992) Sonographic diagnosis of the large for gestational age fetus at term: does it make a difference? *Obstet Gynecol.* **79**: 55–8.

46 Zafeiriou D, Psychogiou K. (2008) Obstetrical brachial plexus palsy. *Pediatr Neurol.* **39**(4): 235–42.

47 Raio L, Ghezzi F, Di Naro E, *et al.* (2003) Perinatal outcome of fetuses with a birth weight greater than 4500g: an analysis of 3356 cases. *Eur J Obstet Gynecol.* **109**: 160–5.

48 Iffy L, Brimacombe M, Apuzzio J, *et al.* (2008) The risk of shoulder dystocia related permanent fetal injury in relation to birth weight. *Eur J Obstet Gynecol Reprod Biol.* **136**(1): 53–60.

49 Irion O, Boulvain M. (2009) Induction of labour for suspected fetal macrosomia (Review). *The Cochrane Collaboration.* Issue 1. London: John Wiley & Sons Ltd.

50 Hankins GDV, Clark SM, Munn MB. (2006) Cesarean section on request at 39 weeks: impact on shoulder dystocia, fetal trauma, neonatal encephalopathy, and intrauterine fetal demise. *Semin Perinatol.* **30**: 276–87.

51 Draycott T, Winter C, Crofts J, Barnfield S, editors. (2008) *PROMPT PRactical Obstetric MultiProfessional Training. Course Manual.* London: RCOG.

52 Boulvain M, Stan C, Irion O. (2001) Elective delivery in diabetic pregnant women. *Cochrane Database Syst Rev.* **2**: CD001997.

53 Gherman RB, Chauhan S, Ouzounian JG, *et al.* (2006) Shoulder dystocia: the unpreventable obstetric emergency with empiric management guidelines. *Am J Obstet Gynecol.* **195**: 657–72.

54 American Academy of Family Physicians. (1996) *Advanced Life Support in Obstetrics.* Newcastle upon Tyne: American Academy of Family Physicians.

55 Gonik B, Zhang N, Grimm MJ. (2003) Prediction of brachial plexus stretching during shoulder dystocia using a computer simulation model. *Am J Obstet Gynecol.* **189**(4): 1168–72.

56 Gherman RB, Tramont J, Muffley P, *et al.* (2000) Analysis of McRoberts' maneuver by x-ray pelvimetry. *Obstet Gynecol.* **95**(1): 43–7.

57 Smeltzer JS. (1986) Prevention and management of shoulder dystocia. *Clin Obstet Gynecol.* **29**(2): 299–308.

58 Gurewitsch ED, Kim EJ, Yang JH, Outland KE, McDonald MK, Allen RH. (2005) Comparing McRoberts' and Rubin's maneuvers for initial management of shoulder dystocia: an objective evaluation. *Am J Obstet Gynecol.* **192**: 153–60.

59 Gherman RB, Ouzounian JG, Incerpi MH, *et al.* (1998) Symphyseal separation and transient femoral neuropathy associated with the McRoberts' maneuver. *Am J Obstet Gynecol.* **178**: 609–10.

60 Heath LT, Gherman RB. (1999) Symphyseal separation, sacroiliac joint dislocation and transient lateral femoral cutaneous neuropathy associated with McRoberts maneuver. *J Reprod Med.* **44**: 902–4.

61 Bruner JP, Drummond SB, Meenan AL, *et al.* (1998) All-fours maneuver for reducing shoulder dystocia during labor. *J Reprod Med.* **43**: 439–43.

62 Kovavisarach E. (2006) The 'all-fours' maneuver for *the* management of shoulder dystocia. *Int J Gynecol Obstet.* **95**(12): 153–4.

63 Naef R, Martin J. (1995) Emergency management of shoulder dystocia. In: Martin J, editor. *Intrapartum and Postpartum Obstetric Emergencies.* Philadelphia, WB Saunders.

64 Gherman RB, Chauhan S, Ouzounian JG, Lerner H, Gonik B, Murphy Goodwin T. (2006) Shoulder dystocia: the unpreventable obstetric emergency with empiric management guidelines. *Am J Obstet Gynecol.* **195**: 657–72.

65 Poggi SH, Spong CY, Allen RH. (2003) Prioritizing posterior arm delivery during severe shoulder dystocia. *Obstet Gynecol.* **101**: 1068–72.

66 Kung J, Swan AV, Arulkumaran S. (2006) Delivery of the posterior arm reduces shoulder dimensions in shoulder dystocia. *Int J Gynecol Obstet.* **93**: 233–7.

68 Gurewitsch ED, Donithan M, Sallings SP, *et al.* (2004) Episiotomy versus fetal manipulation in managing severe shoulder dystocia: a comparison of outcomes. *Am J Obstet Gynecol.* **191**: 911–6.

69 Murphy Goodwin T, Banks E, Millar LK, *et al.* (1997) Catastrophic shoulder dystocia and emergency symphysiotomy. *Am J Obstet Gynecol.* **177**: 463–4.

70 Reid PC, Osuagwu FI. (1999) Symphysiotomy in shoulder dystocia. *J Obstet Gynaecol.* **19**(6): 664–6.

71 Chalidis B, Fahel LA, Glanville T, Kanakaris N, Giannoudis PV. (2007) Management and reconstruction of pelvic instability after emergency symphysiotomy. *Int J Gynecol Obstet.* **98**(3): 264–6.

72 Sandberg EC. (1985) The Zavanelli maneuver: a potentially revolutionary method for the resolution of shoulder dystocia. *Am J Obstet Gynecol.* **152**: 479–84.

73 Namis NN. (1995) Cephalic replacement (the Zavanelli manoeuvre): a desperate solution for severe shoulder dystocia. *Soc Obstet Gynaecol Can.* **17**: 1017–20.

74 Buist R, Khalid O. (1999) Successful Zavanelli manoeuvre for shoulder dystocia with an occipitoposterior position. *Aust N Z J Obstet Gynecol.* **39**(3): 310–11.

75 Sandberg EC. (1999) The Zavanelli maneuver: 12 years of recorded experience. *Obstet Gynecol.* **93**: 312–17.

76 Vollebergh JHA, van Dongen PWJ. (2000) The Zavanelli manoeuvre in shoulder dystocia: case report and review of published cases. *Eur J Obstet Gynecol Reprod Biol.* **89**: 81–4.

77 Smith RB, Lane C, Pearson JF. (1994) Shoulder dystocia: what happens at the next delivery? *Br J Obstet Gynaecol.* **101**: 713–15.

78 Overland EA, Spydslaug A, Nielsen CS, Eskild A. (2009) Risk of shoulder dystocia in second delivery: does a history of shoulder dystocia matter? *Am J Obstet Gynecol.* **200**(5): 506.e1–e6.

79 Moore H, Reed S, Batra M, Schiff M. (2008) Risk factors for recurrent shoulder dystocia. Washington State, 1987–2004. *Am J Obstet Gynecol* **198**: e16.

80 Gurewitsch ED, Johnson TL, Allen RH. (2007) After shoulder dystocia: managing the subsequent pregnancy and delivery. *Semin Perinatol.* **31**: 185–95.

81 Crofts J, Bartlett C, Ellis D, Hunt LP, Fox R, Draycott TJ. (2006) Training for shoulder dystocia: a trial of simulation using low-fidelity and high-fidelity mannequins. *Obstet Gynecol.* **108**(6): 1477–85.

82 Draycott TJ, Ash JF, Wilson JP, Yard LV, Sibanda T, Whitelaw A. (2008) Improving neonatal outcome through practical shoulder dystocia training. *Obstet Gynecol Surv.* **63**(11): 683–4.

83 Heazell AEP, Bhatti NR. (2004) The teaching and use of mnemonic to improve the management of shoulder dystocia. *Clinical Governance: An International Journal.* **9**(4): 253–5.

84 Crofts JF, Bartlett C, Ellis D, Hunt LP, Fox R, Draycott TJ. (2007) Management of shoulder dystocia: skill retention 6 and 12 months after training. *Obstet Gynecol.* **110**(5): 11069–74.

CHAPTER 10

Intrapartum and primary postpartum haemorrhage

Helen Crafter

Introduction

When the usually joyous event of birth is accompanied by excessive bleeding in the mother, the atmosphere in the birth room can change very quickly from being one of calm supportiveness to one of bustling intensity. Yet if the midwife and other health professionals are knowledgeable, well-equipped and confident in their skills, most cases of haemorrhage can be prevented from causing long-term physical damage or emotional trauma to the mother. However, there is no place for complacency. Severe obstetric haemorrhage when it does occur can be lethal and if it does not kill, it can leave women physically damaged and all the family deeply distressed for a very long time. This chapter aims to equip midwives with the knowledge and confidence to prevent and deal with excessive bleeding at and around the time of birth.

Intrapartum haemorrhage (IPH) and primary postpartum haemorrhage (PPH) are commonly defined as excessive blood loss from the genital tract during labour or in the 24 hours following it respectively, of 500 ml or more, or of any amount

that compromises the well-being of the mother. However, these definitions are open to challenge.

Well-nourished pregnant women may lose significantly more blood than 500 ml with no ill effects and before they notice the light-headedness which accompanies acute anaemia. However, this is hardly surprising given that before pregnancy women have a circulating blood volume of approximately four litres and by 30 weeks of gestation this has risen on average by 40%–50%.[1] The definition is perhaps more appropriate to the less well-nourished women of previous decades in the Western world and of women living in poverty today, particularly in poor countries. Most health professionals would argue that it is the woman's overall condition that should indicate to her midwife whether or not she has lost an excessive amount of blood and this will be dictated by her haematological status prior to labour and the events that occur during it. Another problem of defining intrapartum and postpartum blood loss by amount is that it is known that estimation of blood loss at delivery by health professionals is highly inaccurate and becomes more inaccurate the more blood a woman loses.[2,3] In addition blood often remains concealed as a retroplacental clot, or occasionally as intra-abdominal bleeding.[6] Finally, a good midwife does not wait for 500 ml of blood to trickle or gush from the vagina at birth before she acts. If she sees the potential for excessive blood loss unfolding, she acts promptly to try to prevent a haemorrhage or reduce the blood loss. The most important part of the definition of IPH and primary PPH above is therefore 'any amount of blood loss that compromises the well-being of the mother'. However, it should always be borne in mind that compromise to the mother's condition may not be apparent until she has lost a dangerous amount of blood (*see* Table 10.1). This chapter

TABLE 10.1 Maternal symptoms of primary PPH by amount of blood loss (adapted from Mukherjee and Arulkumaran[5])

Average proportion lost of total blood volume (= 6 litres) of a pregnant woman	Amount of blood lost	Degree of shock	Physiological effects	Signs and symptoms a health professional will notice
20%	1200 ml	Mild	Decreased perfusion of non-vital organs and tissues, e.g. bone, fat and skeletal muscle	Pale and cool skin Woman starts to complain of thirst Clamminess Possible mild tachycardia and small drop in blood pressure
20–40%	1200–2400 ml (1500 ml 'potentially life threatening'[7]	Moderate	Decreased perfusion of vital organs and tissues, e.g. gut, liver and kidneys	Skin on legs starts to mottle Tachycardia more noticeable and further drop in blood pressure Oliguria and/or anuria
40% and more	2400 ml+	Severe	Reduced perfusion of heart and brain	Agitation, restlessness, coma Echocardiogram and electrocardiogram abnormalities Metabolic acidosis and finally cardiac arrest

concentrates more on contemporaneous evidence about which actions are effective when a woman bleeds excessively. However, the Cochrane database of systematic reviews advises that treatment for primary PPH need further research.[4]

Incidence of severe obstetric haemorrhage

A study[8] of nearly 50 000 women who gave birth in the South East Thames region over a 12-month period in 1997–98 calculated the severe morbidity rate from obstetric haemorrhage to be 6.7 in every 1000 deliveries, out of a total severe obstetric morbidity rate of 12.0 in every 1000 deliveries. In this study severe haemorrhage was defined as an estimated blood loss of more than 1500 ml, a peripartum fall in haemoglobin concentration of 4 g/dl or an immediate blood transfusion of four or more units of blood.

By any standard these figures suggest that obstetric haemorrhage is a condition requiring the utmost respect from health professionals responsible at birth in understanding the underlying pathology and being knowledgeable and skilful in dealing with such an event.

In the last Report on Confidential Enquiries into Maternal Deaths[9] there were 12 deaths from postpartum haemorrhage, one case of which was a ruptured uterus. Notably, only two of the women were grandmultigravidae, despite this being historically considered as a high-risk category.

In the previous Confidential Enquiries Report[10] it was also suggested that some risk factors for haemorrhage are becoming more common, namely:

- the increasing mean age of childbearing women
- the increasing number of women with complex medical disorders choosing to become pregnant
- an increase in the number of multiple pregnancies following assisted reproduction
- increased caesarean section rate leading to subsequent placenta praevia and accreta.

Causes and predisposing factors

Any combination of the causes (*see* Box 10.1) or predisposing factors (*see* Box 10.2) will increase the risk of IPH and early PPH.

BOX 10.1 Causes

- Placental abruption
- Placenta praevia
- Ruptured uterus
- Cervical or vaginal lacerations
- Atonic uterus, with or without retained products (placenta, membrane and/or blood clot)
- Haematoma.

Note: the woman could display signs of haemorrhage with a less usual site of bleeding, such as subcapsular liver rupture seen in pre-eclampsia and HELLP syndrome.[11]

The main causes of IPH and PPH in Box 10.1, other than atonic uterus and haematoma, are discussed in other chapters so only these two will be addressed in this chapter. The medical predisposing factors also warrant attention because contemporary evidence is increasingly becoming available as to how they affect haemostasis before and after the third stage of labour and how individual conditions should best be managed. Each will be discussed separately here.

BOX 10.2 Physiological/medical predisposing factors

- Raised blood pressure (more than 140/90 mmHg)
- Hydramnios or multiple pregnancy
- Previous caesarean section
- Prolonged labour
- Injudicious use of Syntocinon®
- Precipitate labour
- Supine or semi-recumbent birth
- Instrumental delivery
- Caesarean delivery
- Mismanagement of the third stage of labour
- Morbidly adherent placenta
- Clotting disorder.

It is of note that in the last Confidential Enquiries,[9] of the 17 deaths from haemorrhage, six women were obese and more than half came from ethnic minorities, most of whom spoke no English, and some of whom received no or little antenatal care.

Atonic uterus

Uterine atony remains the most common cause of postpartum haemorrhage.[3]

The uterus literally 'lacks muscle tone' because the myometrium fails to contract and retract as or after the placenta separates. The ruptured blood vessels, common in the normal third stage of labour, at the placental site are not compressed by the living ligature action of the myometrial fibres and bleeding is not controlled. It is worth remembering that in pregnancy at least 500 ml of blood crosses the placenta

every minute[12] and so atony can lead to rapid, heavy blood loss if efficient uterine action is not speedily achieved. Uterine atony is most commonly associated with incomplete separation of the placenta, retained cotyledon, membrane or blood clot, precipitate or prolonged labour, placenta praevia or abruption, general anaesthesia or mismanagement of the third stage. Sometimes its aetiology is unknown. Elizabeth Davis,[13] an American midwife and author, suggests that maternal position may be a factor.

Haematoma

A haematoma is a collection of blood in the tissues which cannot escape – literally a large bruise. Haematomas, when they occur, tend to form in the broad ligament or the lower genital tract during and immediately after birth. A haematoma which forms around the time of birth may occur as a result of a ruptured uterus in labour (*see also* Chapter 8), or ruptured vulval varicose vein in the second stage of labour (*see also* 'Haematoma' in Chapter 12).

Raised blood pressure

Placental abruption is found to be associated in 40% to 50% of women with hypertension in pregnancy; those with hypertension have a five-fold increased risk of abruption.[1] Importantly for the management of maternal haemorrhage either before or after the birth, pre-eclampsia can fulminate rapidly,[14] so a woman presenting with a primary diagnosis of acute haemorrhage may have undiagnosed pre-eclampsia and/or HELPP syndrome. Pre-eclampsia may make her blood pressure soar; haemorrhage may make it plummet. One condition may mask the other so different vital signs must be diligently monitored to effect accurate diagnosis and treatment. For all women presenting in labour with haemorrhage these should include a history of pregnancy and present symptoms, general appearance and condition, pulse, urinalysis and a haematological pre-eclampsia screen (*see* Chapter 4).

Hydramnios or multiple pregnancy

When the membranes rupture in labour in cases of polyhydramnios or following the birth of the first baby in a multiple pregnancy, the sudden and large reduction in the uterine cavity may precipitate placental separation. Where the uterus is overstretched in pregnancy, the muscle cells become less able to contract and retract efficiently in the third stage of labour. The cause of PPH is therefore atonic uterus.

Previous caesarean section

Recent rising caesarean section rates are leading to many questions being asked about the effects on future pregnancy of a uterine scar. The latest two Confidential Enquiries into Maternal Deaths[9,10] acknowledge that in England and Wales there is a rise in cases of placenta praevia and placenta accreta almost certainly due to the rise in caesarean section rates. While awaiting further research, both mothers and birth attendants need to be aware of this risk factor. Caesarean section should therefore be seen in the context of having risk factors for future pregnancies, not just for the present one.

Prolonged labour

Prolonged labour is characterised by weak and incoordinate contractions. Dehydration, ketosis and fatigue may play a part and ultimately uterine muscle will become exhausted.[15] The resulting inertia can lead to uterine atony.

Injudicious use of prostaglandin and Syntocinon®

Prostaglandins and the drug Syntocinon® should be used with great caution. While useful in inducing labour, and preventing excessively long labour and reducing the caesarean section rate when used wisely, imprudent use can damage both the mother and the baby. The use of both prostaglandins and Syntocinon® has been implicated in some cases of uterine rupture in labour, especially if the uterus has been scarred from previous birth or surgery.[9,16] Only one death from genital tract trauma is reported in 2004[10] and one in 2007,[9] both in women who ruptured their uteruses following induction of labour with prostaglandin and precipitate labours. Therefore a good lesson appears to have been learned which should be passed on to students, and must not be forgotten by more experienced practitioners. The 2004 Confidential Enquiry[10] suggests that rupture of the uterus in labour is now so rare that it is prudent for the first consultant obstetrician to call in a second for support (*see also* Chapter 8).

After the birth PPH may occur when a Syntocinon® infusion is stopped as soon as the infant is born and, in the absence of enough naturally produced oxytocin, the relaxed uterine muscle fibres allow excessive passage of blood from the recently separated placental vessels. Therefore Syntocinon® should be discontinued quickly in labour if its use causes problems. However, it should not be discontinued abruptly after the birth of the baby and placenta when uterine muscle relaxation is undesirable.

Precipitate labour

Over-efficiency of the uterus in the first and second stages of labour may lead to failure of retraction of the uterine muscle in the third stage. PPH is the result. Also a speedy passage through the birth canal by the fetus can hinder the gradual and gentle stretching of the tissues, which may lead to lacerations of the cervix, vagina and/or perineum, thereby increasing blood loss.[15]

Supine birth

Elizabeth Davis[13] suggests that if a woman gives birth in an upright position, her abdominal organs will naturally compress her uterus against her pelvic floor. However, if she gives birth in a supine or semi-recumbent position, she is not afforded this advantage. This is one of many choices available to the midwife in aiming to prevent maternal haemorrhage from atony occurring.

Instrumental delivery

Some of the factors which predispose to ventouse and forceps delivery will also predispose to PPH, such as multiple pregnancy, previous caesarean section and prolonged labour, thereby multiplying the risk. Instrumental delivery is also probably a risk factor in itself, as the natural rhythm of labour is countered by an unnaturally expedited birth and the necessity for the uterus to contract and retract immediately. Furthermore, women who have an instrumental delivery will frequently have an episiotomy, which is likely to increase their blood loss. Instrumental delivery also increases the risk of genital tract lacerations.[15,17]

Caesarean delivery

Caesarean birth is almost inevitably associated with a relatively high blood loss because of the amount of tissue incised to reach the baby. Especially in elective surgery maternal oxytocin levels will be low, thereby increasing the risk of atonic uterus, although intravenous Syntocinon® is routinely given to counteract this.

Mismanagement of the third stage

A full bladder in late labour, 'fundus fiddling' (where a health professional applies frequent, irregular pressure to the uterine fundus usually in order to check for good contractility), over-strong cord traction on an unseparated placenta and an inappropriate combination of techniques which should be either actively managed or physiologically managed at the third stage all contribute to incidence of PPH. All interfere with the normal rhythmic contractions which are designed to exactly coordinate muscle contraction and retraction with placental separation, with or without administration of an oxytocic drug.

Morbidly adherent placenta

This refers to placenta accreta, where the placental villi have attached through the decidua into the muscle layer of the uterus; placenta percreta where they have attached through the muscle layer; and the even rarer placenta increta, with attachment right through the muscle layer and encroaching into the perimetrium. PPH occurs when there is partial separation of the placenta, often because only part of the placenta is morbidly adherent, preventing the uterus from contracting adequately.

Clotting disorder

An idiopathic clotting disorder may be present in the mother during pregnancy and its existence may become apparent

---

BOX 10.3 Note on the condition vasa praevia

Vasa praevia is present when there is a velamentous insertion of the umbilical cord into a low-lying placenta. The unprotected fetal blood vessels therefore lie in the lower segment of the uterus, and in front of the presenting part of the fetus. When the membranes rupture, a fetal vessel may also rupture, giving rise to severe fetal bleeding which escapes through mother's vagina. This is not a *maternal* intrapartum haemorrhage; it is the fetus that can exsanguinate, and differentiation between maternal and fetal blood can be difficult.

Vasa praevia is a rare condition, and it is even rarer for a vasa praevia to tear and bleed. A skilled midwife will diagnose the condition with keen, knowledgeable observation and fetal heart rate surveillance. Fetal bleeding starts when the membranes rupture spontaneously or more commonly after their artificial rupture. The midwife will note that the mother will not show any signs of shock but, unless a speedy diagnosis is made and the fetus delivered within minutes, it will die through excessive blood loss.

Although uncommon, occurring in 1:6000 pregnancies, fetal death occurs in 44% of undiagnosed cases. If diagnosed on ultrasound, there is a 97% survival rate for the fetus,[6] but this pre-labour diagnosis is not always available.

---

during routine blood tests, thereby alerting health professionals to an increased risk of bleeding.

Disseminated intravascular coagulopathy (DIC) is an acute condition that occurs when there is a large area of tissue damage, for instance following placental abruption, as a result of pre-eclampsia or eclampsia or following intrauterine fetal death. DIC is very rare when the fetus is alive.[18] A massive release of thromboplastins from the damaged cells into the bloodstream causes widespread clotting throughout the circulation. Clotting factors are used up.[19] Fibrinolysis is triggered and the production of fibrin degradation products (FDPs) further interferes with the process of normal clotting. When no further clotting can take place, uncontrolled bleeding occurs from any site in the body from where blood can escape. (*See* Box 10.9 for information about management and diagnosis of DIC.)

See Box 10.4 for risk reduction measures that can be taken by the midwife.

Diagnosis and management of intrapartum haemorrhage

Vaginal bleeding in the first stage of labour may be due to a show (which can be quite heavy in late labour), placental abruption, placenta praevia or, rarely, a ruptured uterus or vasa praevia. It was noted in a previous Confidential Enquiry in 1998[16] that placenta praevia can remain undiagnosed in pregnancy despite routine and sometimes frequent ultrasound examination.

Resuscitation if required, and diagnosis and management of the cause of bleeding, must be the first priorities in dealing with IPH. It is believed to be good practice for protocols to be in place which give clear instructions about how to deal with major obstetric haemorrhage.[10] The

BOX 10.4 Risk reduction by the midwife

- Encourage an iron rich diet in pregnancy and consider checking haemoglobin levels through later pregnancy so anaemia is avoided as birth approaches.
- Discuss risk and management issues of the third stage of labour in pregnancy and document the woman's wishes (including whether or not she would consent to a blood transfusion, especially if she is a Jehovah's witness, in which case she should have timely antenatal medical review).[3,10]
- Ensure, in particular, women who have had a previous caesarean section are offered an ultrasound scan for placental localisation.
- Know the history of each woman supported in labour. (However, risk assessment in pregnancy does not accurately predict women who will have a PPH.[5])
- Know where all equipment is, especially for emergency procedures.
- Thoroughly understand the pathophysiology of the different causes of bleeding, the signs and symptoms, and the most effective treatments.
- Keep labour as normal as possible by offering good psychological support, non-pharmacological pain relief, information, explanations and a listening ear, and encourage the woman to be as upright and active as she is able.
- Where a woman is likely to benefit from intervention, discuss the benefits and risks with her and her partner and listen to her ideas and concerns, to enhance her feeling of emotional well-being and control.
- Make sure she is as involved in decision making as she is able to be.
- Be aware of the dangers inherent in using prostaglandin, Syntocinon® and mismanaging the third stage of labour.
- Be on good terms with your multiprofessional team. Encourage and if necessary lead the dialogue in decision making. Be prepared to state a case and be an advocate for the woman.
- Ensure that all clinicians are aware of the Unit's protocol for severe obstetric haemorrhage, and ensure it is regularly updated by a multidisciplinary team with obstetric, midwifery, anaesthetic, haematological, radiological and managerial representation.
- Practise 'skills drills' regularly, preferably with the multiprofessional team.

latest CEMACH Report also suggests that resuscitation, and summoning a consultant obstetrician and consultant anaesthetist should be invoked earlier rather than later to **prevent** severe collapse in the mother.[9]

Undiagnosed bleeding in labour

On no account should vaginal examinations or the administration of pessaries, suppositories or enemas be performed until placenta praevia has been categorically ruled out. These procedures can precipitate torrential haemorrhage.

Initial assessment and management of intrapartum haemorrhage

A woman who starts to bleed heavily *per vaginum* in labour will be extremely concerned both for her own safety and that of her baby. As the midwife deals with the situation, either at home or in hospital, her manner and communication skills will be crucial in enlisting the woman's trust and ultimately her cooperation. The feelings of her partner, if present, must also be taken into consideration.

If the woman's medical and pregnancy histories are not available, the midwife should ascertain these as quickly as possible. If she was not present when the bleeding started, she must also find out the circumstances surrounding the blood loss.

Having excluded a normal heavy show in advanced labour, bleeding from haemorrhoids and vasa praevia the midwife must decide whether the woman is having a mild, moderate or severe haemorrhage and on the likely cause. The physiology and management of placental abruption, placenta praevia and ruptured uterus are discussed in Chapters 5 and 8.

As she collects this information the midwife must also carry out observations on the woman. These may include general condition (including pallor, level of consciousness and pain), amount of blood loss, pulse, blood pressure, the nature of any contractions, abdominal girth, abnormal pain (present in between the contractions) and the condition of the fetus. The midwife will be aware that IPH is unpredictable in its course and the woman's condition may deteriorate rapidly with little or no warning. The midwife must therefore decide, while talking to the woman, how urgent the need is for a medical or paramedic presence.

In all cases of IPH at home, it is prudent to agree and arrange immediate transfer to hospital, preferably a maternity unit with an onsite, 24-hour haematology unit and blood bank. The midwife should site an intravenous infusion to access a vein and replace lost fluids. Fluid balance recordings should be commenced.

Having summoned urgent medical aid, and certainly if the labour is being managed in hospital, management of the labour must continue with basic life support if required, resuscitation, appropriate pain relief and a plan for care. If birth is not imminent, caesarean section will be considered.

BOX 10.5 Preparation for immediate delivery by caesarean section

- Maintain resuscitation procedures until surgery.
- Explain to the woman and her partner what is happening and why.
- Maintain frequent observations, record them and share them.
- Inform and involve appropriate personnel, including obstetricians, midwives, the anaesthetist, theatre staff, paediatricians and haematologists.
- Group and cross match blood.
- Routine preparation for surgery, including consent, removal of jewellery and make-up, catheterisation and appropriate local skin care.

Management of haemorrhage after the birth and before delivery of the placenta

Intrapartum haemorrhage after the birth of the baby but before delivery of the placenta is often a midwifery emergency and although medical and senior midwifery aid must be summoned (or emergency services if at home), the situation needs to be dealt with immediately, even while waiting for help. Bleeding may be from the placental site (uterine atony) where the placenta has wholly or partially separated, or from a cervical or vaginal laceration.

The most common predisposing factors for a partially separated placenta include incoordinate action caused by 'fundus fiddling', prolonged labour and precipitate labour.[13] Partial placenta accreta or percreta are also possibilities, although these conditions are rare. Lacerations may complicate any birth, but are more common following compound presentation, birth of a large baby and instrumental delivery.

Bleeding from a laceration is often obvious. If a vessel can be seen spurting or oozing blood it should be immediately clamped and sutured as soon as possible. Occasionally, it is difficult to tell if bleeding is from the uterus, a laceration or both. If the bleeding vessel cannot be located and ligated, and heavy bleeding from the placental bed is suspected, it is prudent to get the placenta delivered as quickly as possible.

Partial separation should be suspected if there is vaginal bleeding with no apparent lengthening of the umbilical cord. Diagnosis is by vaginal examination. If the placenta can be felt just inside the uterine cavity it has separated and should be delivered by controlled cord traction so the cause of the bleeding can be quickly diagnosed and brought under control. However, if the fingers can easily be moved into and up the uterus, partial separation is the most likely cause of bleeding.

If the woman has not recently passed urine, the bladder should be emptied. If she does not have an intravenous infusion with Syntocinon® in place, a bolus of 10 units of intravenous Syntocinon® should be administered and nipple stimulation considered, either by putting the baby to the breast or perhaps by the mother rolling her nipples herself. This will encourage natural oxytocin release within seconds and help the mother to feel she is involved in her own recovery.

Enkin and colleagues[18] report that Syntometrine® is more effective in reducing the risk of PPH than oxytocin alone, although it has more unpleasant side-effects. However Syntocinon® will contract longitudinal fibres only, not the circular ones around the os, and for this reason, if the woman has started to bleed heavily, Syntometrine® or ergometrine which close the os should be avoided before the placenta has delivered.

Of course the reality in modern British obstetrics is that many women will receive Syntometrine® with the birth of the fetal anterior shoulder and the third stage of their labour will then be actively managed to try to ensure that the placenta is delivered within the five to seven minutes before the ergometrine component of the Syntometrine® closes the os. If the placenta remains partially attached and cannot be removed before the os closes, the birth attendants will need to proceed quickly to a manual removal of the placenta, discussed below, to prevent the blood loss becoming excessive. *See* Box 10.7 for a summary of pharmacological management.

Having carried out initial emergency procedures, the midwife should reassess ongoing bleeding and separation of the placenta. If an emergency situation persists and the baby has been born at home, transfer to hospital must be arranged. However, it is always preferable to deliver the placenta before transferring a woman by ambulance and every effort should be made to do so. It is highly dangerous to move a woman who is bleeding heavily from a partially separated placenta.

If it has not already been done, the midwife should now site an intravenous infusion. This must be done before accessible veins in the arms collapse, which would make the procedure more difficult and more time-consuming. Community-based midwives should be proficient in intravenous cannulation and hospital-based midwives will also find it advantageous to have this skill, especially as more birth centres are likely to be set up in the UK in the near future.[20] An intravenous route can then be used to replace lost fluid and may be useful for administering drugs and blood products as necessary.

If bleeding continues, manual removal of the placenta should now be considered (*see* Box 10.6 and Figure 10.1). Although a very simple procedure, it is a painful one for the mother and carries a risk of uterine rupture and infection. Accordingly, the procedure is only suitable in an emergency, although the Midwives Rules and Standards[21] state that

> Member States shall ensure that midwives are at least entitled to take up and pursue . . . the necessary emergency measures in the doctor's absence, in particular manual removal of the placenta, possibly followed by a manual examination of the uterus.

The course of action must be explained to the parents and the partner given the opportunity to leave the room, perhaps to care for the baby, if desired.

> **BOX 10.6** Manual removal of the placenta
> - Observe strict aseptic technique.
> - Use elbow-length gloves.
> - Insert a whole hand (extended) through the os following the cord (if it is still attached to the placenta), while the other hand supports the fundus to prevent it being pushed upwards.
> - Slip the internal hand between the separated portion of the placenta and the wall of the uterus and gently scoop the placenta off with a spatula-like movement, moving the hand smoothly back and forth.
> - Once it has been separated, manually sweep all fragments of placenta from the placental site.
> - Grasp the placenta and manually remove it from the uterus.
> - Once the removal has been completed, the uterus should be vigorously massaged to rub up a contraction.

Syntocinon® should be given, preferably by continuous intravenous infusion, as soon as the placenta is out and this will be continued for a few hours. If the woman is still at home, it may be more appropriate to give ergometrine to aid contraction of the uterus before transfer to hospital. The placenta is quickly examined for completeness, and if there is any doubt an evacuation of the uterus (ERPC) should be considered in hospital. Blood loss must be measured and recorded, and contemporaneous notes made. If she is still at home, the woman should be transferred to hospital whether or not she shows signs

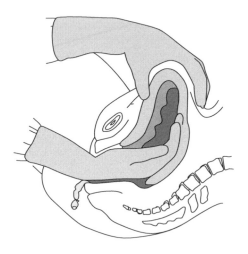

(a) Stage 1: separation

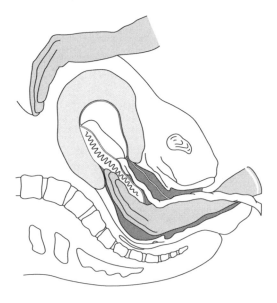

(b) Stage 2: removal

FIGURE 10.1a, b Manual removal of placenta

of shock, in case of uterine muscle relaxation in the next 24 hours. The placenta should also be taken to hospital with the woman, so the obstetricians can make their own decision about its completeness and suggest future management for the woman. She will almost certainly be offered a full blood count to check for anaemia and antibiotics because of her increased risk of uterine infection. Close observation of both the mother and the baby should be continued during this time.

Occasionally, a partially separated placenta cannot be completely removed manually because it is morbidly adherent to the uterine wall. If the midwife suspects this is the case at a home birth, she should administer an oxytocic if there is any blood loss, with the aim of minimising it while transfer to hospital is made.

BOX 10.7 Pharmacological methods of managing atony

Intramuscular, intravenous bolus or intravenous infusion (IVI) of Syntocinon®
Given intramuscularly, Syntocinon® takes 2.5 minutes to act on the uterus and, given intravenously, within 45 seconds. In acute primary PPH, 5 units should be given by slow intravenous injection, followed up by 5–20 more units added to 500 ml intravenous solution and run into the vein at a rate sufficient to control uterine atony. This is the manufacturer's recommended dose, but in practice women may be given up to 50 units in 500 ml of intravenous fluid. Fluid overload must be avoided as this has inherent dangers, particularly adult respiratory distress syndrome (ARDS). High doses

BOX 10.7 (*continued*)

of Syntocinon® can cause nausea, vomiting, arrhythmias, rash and anaphylactic reactions including hypotension.

Intramuscular Syntometrine® (5 units oxytocin and 0.5 mg ergometrine)
Syntometrine® is a drug of choice in British obstetrics as it can be prescribed by the midwife and has a more sustained action than Syntocinon® alone. It will act on the uterus within 2.5 minutes, causing a prolonged contraction. Syntometrine should not be repeated without medical involvement, and no more than two doses in total should be administered because the ergometrine component can cause severe peripheral vasoconstriction, a sharp rise in blood pressure and pulmonary hypertension. For these reasons it should never be administered to women with high blood pressure or severe asthma. It is also contraindicated in women with heart, liver and renal disease and some other medical disorders. Side-effects include nausea and vomiting.

Intramuscular, intravenous bolus or intrauterine injection of ergometrine (0.25–0.5 mg)
Ergometrine can be given intramuscularly, intravenously or directly into uterine muscle. Given intramuscularly, ergometrine takes from 2.5 minutes to act and, given intravenously, up to 45 seconds. If it is injected into uterine muscle it will take effect almost immediately, although this route of administration is rarely seen in practice. A single 0.5 mg dose is recommended for treatment of uterine atony. The same contraindications as for Syntometrine® apply.

Intramuscular carboprost tromethamine (Hemabate®) (250 µg in 1 ml)
Carboprost is a type of prostaglandin that causes contraction of the myometrium to treat atony. It is often given when Syntometrine® and/or Syntocinon® have been ineffective and up to eight doses can be given, no closer than 15 minutes apart and more usually with 1.5 hours between doses. It can potentiate the effect of oxytocin and when both have been used, the woman should be closely monitored. Carboprost should never be given intravenously or to women with hypertension, severe asthma, pelvic inflammatory disease, cardiac, pulmonary, renal or hepatic disease. This drug is not normally accessible at a home birth.

Misoprostol (Cytotec®) (200 microgram oral tablets, 400 microgram rectal, sublingual; can be given vaginally)
Misoprostol is seen on some British delivery suites, and is likely to become increasingly commonly used in both the developed and developing world as it is relatively safe, inexpensive and easy to administer. It tends to be administered rectally at a dose of 400–1000 micrograms for prevention or treatment of PPH, and its efficacy is said to be similar to that of oxytocin, although it can also cause nausea.

Management of haemorrhage after delivery of the placenta

Elizabeth Davis[13] comments that the slow, steady trickle of blood after delivery of the placenta can be the most dangerous of all if it is not closely monitored. Changes of shift, failure to add up the total blood loss and frequent changes of the bed sheets may lead midwives to underestimate the situation and the woman may slowly sink into unconsciousness while the midwife completes her record keeping.

The causes of excessive bleeding after delivery of the placenta tend to be the same as for bleeding before its delivery, namely atonic uterus or lacerations. If there is a continuous gush of blood, the midwife must immediately diagnose the cause of the heavy bleeding. There may or may not have been excessive bleeding before the delivery of the placenta and the present cause of bleeding may or may not remain the same. Continual assessment of the situation is therefore necessary.

Lacerations incurred during the birth of the baby may only now become apparent as a significant cause of bleeding, as expeditious delivery of the placenta may have preoccupied the midwife until now. If the uterus is well contracted, haemostasis needs to be quickly achieved and lacerations sutured. If the woman is at home, the midwife must consider how best to position her and how to achieve optimal lighting, especially if she has not had the opportunity to do this during the woman's pregnancy (for instance in a case of unplanned home birth). This may require some ingenuity on the midwife's part. However, it is vital that the apex of the laceration is identified and repair is undertaken speedily and adequately before the blood loss compromises the well-being of the woman.

If atonic uterus is diagnosed in this situation its cause may remain unknown. However, of the known causes, retention of placental tissue, membrane or blood clot interfering with contraction of the myometrium are the most likely. Retained products can sometimes be diagnosed from examination of the expelled placenta and membranes, but this is by no means foolproof. Clots in the uterus should be suspected if the placenta and membranes appear to be complete, the uterus feels enlarged and a little soft, and a slow trickle of blood after placental delivery gradually increases. A full bladder should also be considered if the bladder has not been emptied recently or the woman has had a high fluid intake (oral or intravenous).

Many predisposing factors to PPH, such as multiple birth, polyhydramnios, antepartum haemorrhage or instrumental delivery will have already led to the attendance of an obstetrician. However, if uterine atony is diagnosed and a doctor is not present, the midwife should immediately summon medical aid, explain what is happening to the woman and her birth partner, tell them briefly what she is going to do and ask for their cooperation. The woman needs to get into a semi-recumbent or recumbent position preferably on a bed. The uterus should be made to contract as soon as possible by the following means.

- Rub up a contraction (*see* Box 10.8 and Figure 10.2). This should also express retained blood clots.
- Catheterise the bladder. Any urine contained may interfere with strong contraction and at this point the midwife needs to know that the bladder is empty and kept empty until the bleeding is brought under control.

- Consider a (further) dose of Syntocinon® as an intravenous bolus or by infusion, or Syntometrine® intramuscularly (if not contraindicated). If the woman is able to put the baby to the breast this will release natural oxytocin, which will promote uterine muscle contraction.

These measures will bring most cases of haemorrhage from atony speedily under control. However, if bleeding is becoming potentially life-threatening, the midwife should perform bi-manual compression (*see* Figure 10.3).

To achieve bi-manual compression one hand is placed in the anterior fornix of the vagina and clenched, while the other hand massages the fundus, thereby pressing the walls of the uterus together.

BOX 10.8 Rubbing up a contraction

- Gently feel for the fundus with the pads of the fingertips (a manoeuvre similar to palpation of the fundus in pregnancy) and assess uterine contraction. A right-handed midwife standing on the woman's right side will do this with the left hand.
- Cup the hand around the uterus and massage it firmly but gently (this action should not be overly painful for the woman) with a smooth, circular movement until its soft texture starts to become firmer with an oncoming contraction.
- Hold the hand still and do not recommence massage unless the uterus starts to relax again.

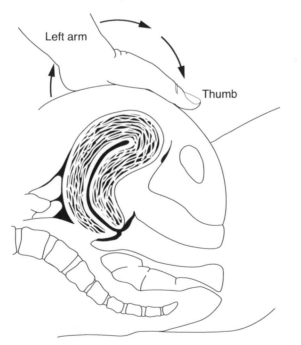

Left arm

Thumb

The left hand is cupped over the uterus ( ) and massages it with a firm circular motion in a clockwise direction.

FIGURE 10.2 Rubbing up a contraction

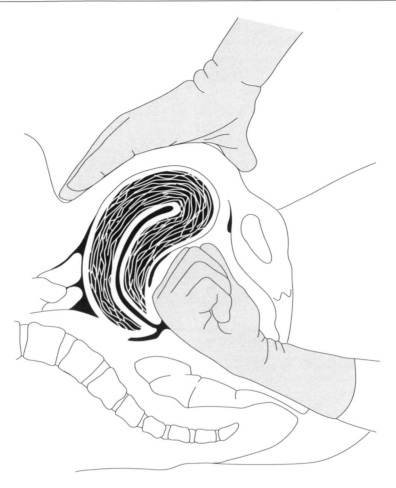

FIGURE 10.3 Internal bi-manual compression

Alternatively, bi-manual compression can be done externally by grasping the uterus with both hands and squashing the uterus between them.[13] It should be noted that internal bi-manual compression in particular is extremely painful for the woman and should only be performed if other procedures are not effective, while awaiting medical action. Needless to say all this should be explained clearly to the woman and her partner before the procedure is attempted, as great distress will be caused if either is unprepared for the extreme discomfort which will ensue.

If these procedures do not work, the midwife and any other health professionals who have been summoned should consider a blood coagulation problem. Urgent blood tests will be done to enable diagnosis and the correct management. The mother is now likely to be shocked and should be treated with intravenous fluids and appropriate drugs. A central venous line may be indicated and a blood transfusion ordered. Bi-manual compression will need to be continued until the bleeding is brought under control.

A blood coagulation problem is relatively easy to diagnose because bleeding continues either in a steady stream or a gush and does not clot where it collects. Once medical diagnosis has been made and haematological results are known to ascertain the extent of the problem, it can be treated accordingly.

In all cases of continued bleeding, uterine packing (tamponade) may be considered.[3,15,22] Dry sterile gauze is used, which can be moistened with saline. Analgesia is required during the procedure and antibiotic cover is suggested.

A bladder catheter should remain *in situ* for 24–36 hours until the pack is removed on the delivery suite, with operating facilities at the ready in case bleeding restarts. A danger is that an obstetrician may pack the uterus to arrest the bleeding when unable to diagnose the cause; in such a case laparotomy, to discover and then treat the actual cause, may be safer. However, uterine packing can be a useful measure while a woman is transferred to an operating theatre for more intensive treatment.

Less common treatments, which have been attempted with varying success in

---

BOX 10.9 Diagnosis and management of disseminated intravascular coagulopathy

Diagnosis

- An acute history of a predisposing condition (e.g. placental abruption)
- Bleeding from orifices, e.g. nose, mouth, venepuncture site, haematuria
- Blood loss does not immediately clot
- Torrential haemorrhage
- Signs of circulatory obstruction, e.g. cyanosis in fingers, cerebrovascular accident (stroke) or renal failure
- Blood test results: low haemoglobin, abnormal clotting study results (prothrombin time, abnormal levels of platelets, fibrinogen and FDPs)
- Prompt diagnosis and management are vital for maternal survival.

Management

- Refer to the local protocol, which should be drawn up on how DIC should be managed.
- Request urgent medical attendance when DIC is suspected.
- Look for the underlying cause if it is not known (DIC is never a primary disease), although the woman's condition will need to be stabilised before the condition is treated (or the baby delivered, when the condition occurs in pregnancy).
- Give explanations and emotional support to the woman and her partner as necessary.
- Urgent blood test results will dictate the course of management, including full blood count, clotting studies and time taken to group and cross match blood. Replacement of blood cells and clotting factors will be required with fresh frozen plasma, platelet concentrates and, ultimately, with red blood cells.
- Maintain frequent and accurate observations of the woman's vital signs. Invasive monitoring with a central venous pressure and/or arterial line may be necessary. The bladder should be catheterised and fluid balance vigilantly monitored. Any sign of renal failure must be reported to the team immediately.

the control of PPH and in which the midwife may be called upon to assist the medical practitioner, include bilateral internal iliac artery ligation, bilateral uterine artery ligation, bilateral ovarian and uterine artery ligation, arterial occlusion or embolisation, applying haemostatic (compression: brace or B-Lynch) sutures or insertion of a balloon catheter into the uterus (balloon tamponade).[3,22] Hysterectomy is a final resort.

Uterine artery embolisation appears to be an increasingly adopted procedure in the UK and although this appears to be an effective way of avoiding hysterectomy in intractable haemorrhage with a more than 95% success rate,[22] the necessity of performing the procedure under radiological guidance makes it impractical in many maternity units.

Unusually, a postpartum haemorrhage may present as a *haematoma*, concealed in the broad ligament or the vaginal wall. Up to 1 litre of blood can collect in the tissues.[15] Symptoms include pain at the site, collapse and shock, and it can be seen on ultrasound. The woman should be transferred to the operating theatre where the haematoma should be drained and haemostasis achieved under spinal or epidural anaesthesia. Blood replacement may be required, and antibiotics should be given.

Once the bleeding has been controlled the woman must be carefully observed, and her recovery carefully managed, possibly in either a high-dependency unit on the delivery suite or in an intensive care unit. The needs of all the family should also continue to be met.

As with all midwifery actions, record keeping is important and notes should be kept as contemporaneously as possible.

Conclusion

Peripartum haemorrhage in the mother is the obstetric emergency the midwife is most likely to face in her career. Many potential cases can be and are avoided by skilled support of women throughout pregnancy and in labour. Some cases can be predicted from women's histories and with the appropriate use of technology, but most cases are unforeseen and their course is unpredictable. Wherever possible, management options should be discussed with the woman to ensure that she is involved in decision making about her care. As most cases of obstetric haemorrhage occur without warning the midwife, along with the multiprofessional obstetric team, needs to be continually vigilant, and equipped to deal with these situations whether at home, in a birth centre or in hospital.

With prompt and skilful management, the majority of intrapartum and early postpartum haemorrhages can be brought under control with a minimum of interventions. However, in the latest Confidential Enquiries published in 2007,[9] 58% of the 19 maternal deaths for postpartum haemorrhage included one or more elements of substandard care; this suggests that we all still have many lessons to learn.

References

1 Francois KE, Foley MR. (2007) Antepartum and postpartum haemorrhage. In: Gabbe SG, Neibyl JR, Simpson JL, editors. *Obstetrics Normal and Problem Pregnancies*. 5th ed. Philadelphia: Churchill Livingstone Elsevier. pp. 456–85.

2 Davis K, Rucklidge M. (2007) Management of obstetric haemorrhage. Anaesthesia UK. Available at: www.frca.co.uk/article.aspx?articleid=100758 (accessed 8 June 2009).

3   Royal College of Obstetricians and Gynaecologists (RCOG). (2009) *Prevention and Management of Postpartum Haemorrhage. Green-top Guideline No. 52.* London: RCOG.

4   Mousa HA, Alfirevic Z. (2007) Treatment for primary postpartum haemorrhage. *Cochrane Database Syst Rev.* **1**: CD003249.

5   Mukherjee S, Arulkumaran S. (2009) Postpartum haemorrhage. *Obstet Gynaecol Reprod Med.* **19**(5): 121–6.

6   Mukherjee S, Bhide A. (2008) Antepartum haemorrhage. *Obstet Gynaecol Reprod Med.* **18**(12): 335–9.

7   PRactical Obstetric MultiProfessional Training (PROMPT). (2008): *Module 8: major obstetric haemorrhage.* London: RCOG Press.

8   Waterstone M, Bewley S, Wolfe C. (2001) Incidence and predictors of severe obstetric morbidity: case control study. *BMJ.* **322**: 1089–94.

9   Lewis G, editor. (2007) *Saving Mothers Lives 2003–2005. Seventh Report on Confidential Enquiries into Maternal Deaths in the United Kingdom.* London: CEMACH.

10 Lewis G, Drife J, editors. (2004) *Why Mothers Die 2002–2004. The Sixth Report of Confidential Enquiries into Maternal Deaths in the United Kingdom.* London: RCOG Press.

11 Williamson C, Girling J. (2007) Hepatic and gastrointestinal disease. In: James DK, Steer PJ, Weiner CP, Gonik B, editors. *High Risk Pregnancy: management options.* Philadelphia: WB Saunders. pp. 1032–60.

12 Stables D. (1999) *Physiology of Childbearing.* London: Baillière Tindall.

13 Davis E. (1997) *Hearts and Hands.* Berkeley: Celestial Arts.

14 Boyce T, Dodd C, Waugh J. (2008) Hypertensive disorders. In: Robson SE, Waugh J, editors. *Medical Disorders of Pregnancy: a manual for midwives.* Chichester: Blackwell Publishing. pp. 19–26.

15 Ndala R. (2005) Postpartum haemorrhage and other third-stage problems. In: Stables D, Rankin J, editors. *Physiology in Childbearing.* 2nd ed. Edinburgh: Elsevier. pp. 575–84.

16 Department of Health. (1998) *Why Mothers Die: report on confidential enquiries into maternal deaths in the United Kingdom 1994–1996.* London: The Stationery Office.

17 Evans W, Edelstone DI. (2000) Instrumental delivery. In: Kean LH, Baker PN, Edelstone DI, editors. *Best Practice in Labour Ward Management.* Edinburgh: WB Saunders.

18 Enkin M, Keirse MJNC, Neilson J, *et al.* (2000) *A Guide to Effective Care in Pregnancy and Labour.* Oxford: Oxford University Press.

19 Crafter H. (2009) Problems of pregnancy In: Fraser DM, Cooper MA, editors. *Myles Textbook for Midwives.* Edinburgh: Elsevier. pp. 333–60.

20 Rosser J. (2001) Birth centres across the UK: a win/win strategy for saving normal birth. *RCM Midwives.* **4**(3): 88–9.

21 Nursing and Midwifery Council (NMC). (2004) *Midwives Rules and Standards.* London: UKCC.

22 Rogers MS, Chang AMZ. (2007) Postpartum haemorrhage and other problems of the third stage. In: James DK, Steer PJ, Weiner CP, Gonik B, editors. *High Risk Pregnancy: management options.* 3rd ed. Philadelphia: WB Saunders. pp. 1559–78.

CHAPTER 11

Amniotic fluid embolism (anaphylactoid syndrome of pregnancy)

Maureen Boyle

Amniotic fluid embolism (AFE) is an obstetric emergency that is impossible to predict, offers minimal, if any, warning signs and frequently has a tragic outcome. Internationally, in all countries which keep comprehensive records, AFE is identified as one of the most significant contributors to maternal mortality, accounting for 10% of all maternal deaths in Australia[1] and 7.5% in the USA.[2] In the UK, the latest Confidential Enquiries into Maternal Deaths[3] has identified AFE as the second highest obstetric reason for women to die, recording 0.80 per 100 000 maternities. This finding comes after several trienniums where, apart from 1994–96 where the rate was 0.77 per 100 000 maternities, numbers ranged between 0.25 and 0.40. There seems to be no clear reason for this sudden jump, but better recognition of the condition, and improved pathological investigation, may have contributed to correct attribution. However, as the deaths were not spread evenly through the three years, it cannot be assumed that these findings represent a consistent trend.[3]

Amniotic fluid embolism is difficult to diagnose, especially when the outcome is not fatal. The most often quoted occurrence rates are anywhere from 1:8000 to 1:80 000, the UK incidence 1.8:100 000[4] or 1:120 000.[2] A mortality rate of up to 90% is still suggested in some literature, although recent American studies[5–8] showed maternal mortality rates of 13%–30%. In the UK there is a suggested rate of 37% mortality[9] and case analysis has shown that 25% of women die in the first hour, and most of the others by nine hours.[2] However, significant long-term morbidity is frequently associated with AFE,[2] and for those babies who were undelivered when their mothers suffered AFE, significant morbidity was also noted.

An early description of amniotic fluid embolism was made in 1941 as 'maternal pulmonary embolism by amniotic fluid', after finding amniotic fluid in the pulmonary vessels at post mortem, following a collapse during delivery with symptoms mimicking pulmonary embolism.[10] Knowledge of the condition has only developed slowly since then, due to its rarity. However, in 1988 a central registry recording women suffering from amniotic fluid embolism in the USA was set up and reports from this group have contributed to awareness.[11] In the UK, a similar registry was set up in 2000,[12] and collection of data is now under the umbrella of the UK Obstetric Surveillance System (UKOSS), their latest report on AFE being in 2007.[4] Now investigation has been taken over by UKOSS it is likely the number identified will grow – in 18 months from February 2005 to July 2006, 19 cases were confirmed.[3]

Pathophysiology

AFE is now seen as a maternal response to the amniotic fluid and/or fetal debris in her circulation, rather than the fluid itself causing a blockage, and this is represented in the suggested new name: anaphylactoid syndrome of pregnancy (various other names have also been suggested, such as 'anaphylactoid lung of pregnancy'[13] and 'sudden obstetric collapse syndrome'.[9])

Amniotic fluid can enter the maternal circulation through the endocervical veins and it is suggested that it may do so frequently without damage, although others disagree,[9,14] arguing that the diagnostic squamous cells may be maternal rather than fetal. Evidence for this has been when squames have been observed in blood taken from non-pregnant women in specimens from pulmonary artery catheters.[14] It has been observed that pregnant women with clinical signs of AFE have mucin, lanugo, vernix and/or meconium present in blood from their pulmonary circulation, and these are often coated with leukocytes, which could indicate that this fetal debris caused a maternal reaction.[1,11] It has also been noted that if meconium or an intrauterine death is present, the time from the first presentation of symptoms to cardiac arrest and

death is shorter than when clear liquor is present.[11]

Although amniotic fluid may be able to enter the maternal circulation without causing problems, in some women it seems an inflammatory response can develop, causing a rapid collapse similar to anaphylaxis or septic shock.[15] One suggestion is that amniotic fluid in the maternal circulation could result in the release of a substance (endothelin[16,17] has been suggested) which leads to pulmonary vascular spasm, which in turn causes left ventricular failure. Others have suggested that bioactive chemicals present in the amniotic fluid cause these reactions directly.[14] Pulmonary vasoconstriction and increased pulmonary vascular resistance may cause the cardiovascular collapse, and this may in turn result in later left ventricular failure. There may also be a direct myocardial depression by the amniotic fluid (or other factors).[5]

It has also been suggested that an immune reaction may be triggered by fetal antigens, resulting in activation of the complement system.[18] However, specific causes are still unknown – it may be that it is the amount of amniotic fluid, the chemical composition or the individual woman's susceptibility that causes the AFE, or perhaps a combination of these or other unknown factors.

AFE is a rare occurrence, but why some women are susceptible and others are not is unknown. The suggestion that an anaphylactic-type reaction is the cause of the symptoms is supported by findings that suggest women with a history of atopy and allergy appear at more risk.[6]

Obvious times of risk for entry of amniotic fluid and its constituents are during caesarean section or uterine rupture, but since amniotic fluid embolism can occur without these scenarios, it is also suggested that there may be small injuries during labour that allow the fluid access to maternal circulation. Amniotomy is an intervention that may cause injury and it has been reported that in the American Registry 78% of women with amniotic fluid embolism had ruptured membranes (two-thirds being artificial rupture of membranes: ARM).[12] In 13% of cases only three minutes separated the ARM or insertion of intrauterine pressure catheters (IUPCs) and the maternal collapse. However, it is clear that in some cases the damage may occur spontaneously. A recent finding that placenta praevia and placenta abruption may be predisposing factors for AFE[6] is a further indication that the breakdown of the maternal/fetal barrier may be significant.

The volume of amniotic fluid entering the maternal circulation does not seem relevant, as AFE has been diagnosed during termination of early pregnancy, when there is only a very small amount of fluid present.[19]

Although the exact underlying pathophysiology and the reasons why any individual women might be susceptible are not completely understood, the physical effects are clear. The pulmonary circulation is compromised, right and left ventricular failure may occur, and coronary artery vasospasm may cause myocardial ischaemia. However, it may be that individual women exhibit different processes, although the results may be the same.

Secondary coagulation problems affect most women developing AFE.[17] The cause of this coagulopathy is not well understood, but one suggestion is that disseminated intravascular coagulation may be due to amniotic fluid activating the extrinsic pathway, thereby triggering clotting and the development of a consumptive coagulopathy.[5] It is known that amniotic fluid is a procoagulant, but this may not be enough to cause the often catastrophic haemorrhage.[9] The coagulopathy may also be a result of complementary activation, not a response to pre-coagulation.[18] It has been noted that there may be increased coagulation pathology when meconium is present.[17]

Although many definitions describe the timing of AFE restricted to occurrence in labour and immediately post delivery, there are cases that have been reported after first trimester termination, amniocentesis,[20,21] in the second trimester,[22] after trauma[23] and postnatally.[24]

There have also been reports of amniotic fluid embolism occurring later than would be expected, for example following caesarean section rather than during the procedure. It is suggested that such a delayed reaction may occur following a spinal anaesthesia if the amniotic fluid is present in dilated uterine veins and this is displaced when the block wears off and the venous tone is allowed to return.[25] Additionally, there have been rare reports of AFE occurring up to 48 hours post delivery, and the suggestion was made that amniotic fluid and fetal debris in uterine veins moved into the circulation only during involution of the uterus.[5]

Diagnosis

Historically, diagnosis of amniotic fluid embolism was only made on post mortem examination when fetal cells or debris were found during histological analysis of the maternal lungs.[26] Diagnosis has also been made in women who have survived, for example, following special staining of blood from the mothers' pulmonary vessels[7] or after finding fetal squames in sputum. However, these cells may be due to contamination, and adult and fetal squames cannot be distinguished histologically.[9] Of course these tests are usually carried out only when the mother's physical condition is compromised. It should also be noted that evidence of fetal debris in maternal lungs may not be present at post mortem if she had survived for several days.[9]

Diagnosis of amniotic fluid embolism through analysis of maternal serum has been suggested. Although assessment of serum tryptase levels (an indication of a low complement)[27] has been suggested to be useful,[9] these have so far been proven to be inconclusive.[17] Elevated levels of fetal antigen sialyl Tn, a constituent of amniotic fluid and meconium[28] and zinc coproporphyrin (a component of meconium)[29] have also been suggested as substances which could be assessed to aid diagnosis.

However, at present, most authorities agree that diagnosis should be made on the basis of clinical signs and symptoms. Clark[15] described the sudden onset of a triad of symptoms, namely *hypotension*, *hypoxia* and *coagulopathy*, as highly suspicious. Amniotic fluid embolism should always be suspected if a previously asymptomatic healthy woman develops cardiac or respiratory failure during labour, caesarean section or immediately after.[3,30]

Investigations which may aid diagnosis by excluding other possible conditions include *chest X-rays* (usually non-specific in AFE but may show pulmonary oedema if present),[31] *12-lead ECG* (which may show changes from right ventricular strain), *echocardiograms* (may confirm right or left ventricular failure), *lung V/Q scan* (may show non-specific perfusion defects) and *blood tests* (in particular clotting which may demonstrate

coagulopathy). However, no tests should delay basic, comprehensive and ongoing resuscitation: The Confidential Enquiries[3] notes substandard care in two cases where resuscitation was delayed as women were sent for unnecessary diagnostic scans.

Signs and symptoms

The first symptoms seen may be shortness of breath, altered mental status and agitation,[13] followed by cardiovascular collapse and DIC.[32] However, there are many reports of other signs and symptoms presenting first: 10%–20% of those with AFE may have haemorrhage or convulsions as their first symptoms.[9] Tuffnell[33] reported a sudden deterioration of the fetal heart rate in 36% of cases.

The analysis of the American Registry showed that the symptoms of women diagnosed with amniotic fluid embolism were as follows, given in the order in which they most commonly occurred:[11]

- hypotension
- fetal distress
- pulmonary oedema
- cardiopulmonary arrest
- cyanosis
- coagulopathy
- respiratory distress
- convulsions
- uterine atony
- bronchospasm.

However, in individual women, these symptoms can appear alone, in combination and of course in any order. Ten to 15% of women may have seizures as the first sign of amniotic fluid embolism, obviously causing the potential for confusion with eclampsia.[34]

There is a suggestion that women presented with vague 'premonitory' signs and symptoms, such as breathlessness, chest pain, light-headedness, nausea/vomiting, distress or panic immediately or up to four hours prior to AFE.[3] While these may be frequently reported in notes of those prior to an AFE, none is an unknown symptom to experienced labour ward midwives. Breathlessness and chest pain will of course be immediately referred as appropriate, but in general all these signs and symptoms are common in active labour, especially when approaching the second stage. It will be challenging for the midwife to distinguish the normal from the abnormal.

Predisposing/risk factors

A condition which is rare, and where the understanding of the pathophysiology is so uncertain, is a difficult one for which to establish clear predisposing and risk factors. However, many have been identified, although some are controversial (*see* Box 11.1 for a summary).[6,9,35] Induction with prostaglandins or oxytocin, or augmentation with oxytocin or artificial rupture of membranes (ARM), are often considered to be associated with amniotic fluid embolism. Medical induction has been said to increase the risk of AFE.[36] However, in the Confidential Enquiries,[3] of the 17 women who died, eight had received uterine stimulation (three oxytocin, five prostaglandins), and two had received artificial rupture of membranes. The role of induction and augmentation is therefore far from clear.

'Tumultuous' labour was described in 28% of women in one American report[34] and abnormally strong contractions have also been noted by previous Confidential Enquiries in the UK.[26] If the strength of contractions is considered to have influence over the occurrence of amniotic fluid

> **BOX 11.1** Predisposing/risk factors for AFE
> - Age >35
> - Multiparity
> - Multiple pregnancy/large fetus (uterine overdistension)
> - Pre-eclampsia/eclampsia
> - Polyhydramnious
> - Abruption/placenta praevia
> - Induction/augmentation of labour
> - 'Tumultuous' contractions
> - Meconium
> - Long labour
> - Fetal distress
> - Invasive interventions in labour
> - Caesarean section
> - Instrumental delivery
> - Uterine rupture.

embolism, multiparous women could be assumed to have very strong contractions and therefore be at increased risk. Out of 17 maternal mortalities for amniotic fluid embolism in the UK reported in the years 2003–05, 13 had a history of one or more previous deliveries.[3] It is also possible that the reported tumultuous contractions are not associated with the reason the AFE occurs but they are a reaction to it. It is a common characteristic of mammals when a sudden threatening pathophysiological event occurs for the body to make a desperate attempt to rid itself of the pregnancy in order to survive. This could be a normal reaction of the woman's body to try to survive the acute insult of the AFE.

There appears to be an association between amniotic fluid embolism and operative or instrumental deliveries, and with any invasive interventions such as amniotomy, insertion of IUPCs and amnioinfusion. It has been noted that

78% of women first demonstrated symptoms of AFE after rupture of membranes (both spontaneous and artificial) and insertion of an IUPC.[9] Caesarean section is particularly noted in the most recent large American study,[6] but the most common associations were placenta praevia, abruption and 'elderly primigravidae'.

Amniotic fluid embolism appears to be more common with increasing age. The Report on Confidential Enquires into Maternal Deaths[3] identified that in the years 2003–05 the median age was 33 years. Interestingly, in a large recent study (almost 3 million hospital records over five years reviewed), 'elderly primiparous' women were significantly more likely to suffer AFE.[6] However, there were no deaths in this category. This is particularly relevant as it is assumed this group would be more likely to have induction of labour, caesarean section and other interventions, and therefore have multiple risk factors. Could it be the increased surveillance led to quicker recognition and treatment, and therefore a better outcome?

Although the roles of different risk factors are uncertain, they do serve to highlight the range of women who may suffer AFE, and the necessity for the midwife to keep the possibility of an occurrence in mind.

Treatment

Since it is not yet possible to clearly identify those women who are at risk of amniotic fluid embolism or to prevent it, the focus must be on providing any woman who collapses with prompt and competent first aid prior to a speedy transfer to where she can receive expert support and care, usually in an intensive care unit. This can improve her chance not only of survival, but of a complete recovery. General aims of treatment are given in Box 11.2.

BOX 11.2 Treatment aims
- Circulatory support
- Respiratory support
- Correct coagulopathy.

Initial care

This will be the same whether at home or in hospital and includes the following:
- Call for emergency help
- Intravenous access and fluids
- Ventilation: oxygen administration, mouth to mouth, manual ventilation with an ambubag or intubation, depending on the site and availability of equipment or personnel
- Cardiac massage as necessary.

(*See* Chapter 2 for further detail of basic resuscitation.)

Ongoing care

Following the arrival of help in hospital or the woman's arrival at hospital, the priorities of care given in Box 11.2 continue:
- Administer fluids to maintain circulation (may be blood, fresh frozen plasma, cryoprecipitates, crystalloids or platelets depending on availability and the woman's need). Fluids are given to maintain blood pressure and respond to haemorrhage – note, however, that there is a danger of overload, leading to pulmonary oedema, so careful records need to be maintained.
- Monitor clotting and correct coagulopathy.

- Early endotracheal intubation as necessary.
- Maintain oxygenation via intermittent positive pressure ventilation (IPPV) as necessary.
- Monitor condition, initially with pulse oximetry and cardiac monitor, then central venous pressure, arterial lines or pulmonary artery catheters as appropriate. Coagulopathy may restrict the ability to use invasive monitoring.
- Careful fluid balance and renal assessment (including early insertion of an indwelling urinary catheter).
- Deliver the baby if necessary to enable efficient resuscitation.
- Maintain uterine tone if necessary – initially with bi-manual compression, then surgically (packing, tamponade, balloon, brace suture, hysterectomy) or medically (oxytocics, ergometrine, prostaglandins).
- Administer drugs as necessary:
  – dopamine (increases cardiac output)
  – hydrocortisone (reduces inflammatory response)
  – sodium bicarbonate (corrects acidosis).

The literature has reported various therapies, including high-dose corticosteroids, epinephrine,[11] serine protease inhibitors and nitric oxide.[37] It is unlikely there will ever be any clear evidence on which is the best, until more is known about the cause and pathophysiology of AFE.

There have also been reports in the literature of recombinant activated factor VIIa being used successfully in some cases to reverse DIC.[38] Other less common treatment such as cardiopulmonary bypass has been described[39] but, as for all treatments, success will be dependent on early recognition of the condition and effective resuscitation.

Support and care for partners and others must not be neglected (*see* Chapter 2 and 13 for further discussion on this important matter) and consideration of psychological support for women who survive is necessary.

Complications

Of women who collapse with amniotic fluid embolism, 25%–50% may die within the first hour.[30] A recent review suggested that the women who died did so within seven hours of their collapse.[40] The most common short-term complication of amniotic fluid embolism is DIC, arising in around half of those who survive more than one hour.[30] Many survivors have permanent neurological damage and neurologically intact survival has been estimated at only about 15%;[41] however, with better recognition and care this number should be rising significantly.

If the woman is still pregnant when suffering the amniotic fluid embolism, the fetus may not survive. Estimates of fetal survival rates range from 39% to 80%. In the most recent Confidential Enquiries,[3] apart from the three babies who were born before their mothers' collapse, 10 out of 16 babies survived, including one-third of babies delivered by peri or post-mortem caesarean section. It has, however, been suggested that even if the baby lives, neurological damage to the infant is common.[11]

Although there is little in the literature about further pregnancies after a woman has survived an AFE, it is suggested a repeat occurrence is unlikely[42] and successful pregnancies have been reported.[43]

Midwifery considerations following maternal collapse

- Instigate resuscitation and summon team (major obstetric emergency).
- Cannulate (two large-bore cannulae if possible) and catheterise.
- Commence pulse oximetry and three-lead ECG monitoring.
- Be able to access all emergency drugs and appropriate equipment.
- Assist anaesthetist in respiratory support as necessary.
- Liaise with blood bank and haematologist.
- Administer fluids including all blood products as prescribed.
- If caesarean section is necessary to enable more efficient resuscitation, coordinate paediatric services.
- If the baby was born before the collapse, ensure he/she is appropriately cared for.
- Ensure partner and other family/friends present are informed and given support as appropriate (*see* Chapters 2 and 13).
- Ensure accurate and contemporaneous records are kept, including personnel attending, actions taken, fluids and drugs administered and vital signs.

Conclusion

It is not possible to clearly identify how to prevent amniotic fluid embolism. However, it still seems clear that care needs to be taken in the use of prostaglandins and oxytocins, particularly in those women with other possible risk factors, for example age, parity and obstetric complications, and that other obstetric interventions, such as amniotomy, should be used only when necessary.

The Confidential Enquiries reports have recommended that better treatment for those women that survive the initial event may help improve the outcome. Lewis[3] identified substandard care in seven (36%) cases. Some deaths may have been inevitable, but delay in starting resuscitation was noted in most. For two of the women, midwifery care may be distinctly identified – drugs and equipment were not easily accessible and the arrest team could not gain entry to the labour ward. There was also a case of a woman who had identified that she would refuse blood products, but there was no advanced care plan in her notes.

Labour, and especially transition, is often a time of mood change and uncharacteristic maternal behaviour, and midwives are very familiar with this scenario. However, given that confusion and/or behaviour/mood change can be the first sign of hypoxia, if the midwife can assess this quickly with a saturation reading, she can be reassured – or in the unlikely event hypoxia is present, summon help immediately, ensuring as early action as possible is obtained. Until there is further knowledge of the meaning and reliability of these noted 'premonitory' signs, there seems little else the midwife can do other than ensure she is alert.

All units should have regular 'skills drills' and it should be mandatory for all those working to update regularly – emergencies happen too infrequently for any midwife or doctor to be complacent about their abilities. It is also particularly useful (although admittedly challenging to arrange) if at least some of these take place on the labour ward itself, which could help to ensure all personnel knew how to access relevant drugs and equipment and that the arrest team could gain easy access through security doors etc.

Key points of midwifery care

- Use midwifery skills to augment slow labour (e.g. support, mobilisation, comfort strategies, etc.) to avoid amniotomy and oxytocin use.
- Despite their common use, always treat prostaglandin and oxytocin with respect and monitor all women receiving these drugs carefully to avoid overstimulation. Use particular care when administering to older women, multiparous women or those with other complications.
- If a woman collapses at home or in hospital, prompt effective emergency support can improve her chance of complete recovery.

References

1 Burrows A, Khoo S. (1995) The amniotic fluid embolism syndrome: 10 years' experience at a major teaching hospital. *Aust N Z J Obstet Gynaecol.* **35**: 245–50.
2 Tuffnell D. (2005) United Kingdom Amniotic Fluid Embolism Register. *Br J Obstet Gynaecol.* **112**: 1625–9.
3 Lewis G, editor. (2007) *The Confidential Enquiry into Maternal and Child Health (CEMACH). Saving Mothers' Lives: reviewing maternal deaths to make motherhood safer 2003–2005. The Seventh Report on Confidential Enquiries into Maternal Deaths in the UK.* London, CEMACH.
4 Knight M, Kurinczuk J, Spark P, Brocklehurst P. (2007) *United Kingdom Obstetric Surveillance System (UKOSS) Annual Report.* Oxford: National Perinatal Epidemiology Unit.
5 Conde-Agudelo A, Romero R. (2009) Amniotic fluid embolism: an evidence-based review. *Am J Obstet Gynecol.* **201**(5): 445–55.
6 Abenhaim H, Azoulay L, Kramer M, Leduc L. (2008) Incidence and risk factors of amniotic fluid embolisms: a population-based study of 3 million births in the United States. *Am J Obstet Gynecol.* **199**(49): 49–52.
7 Locksmith G. (1999) Amniotic fluid embolism. *Obstet Gynecol Clin North Am.* **26**(3): 435–44.
8 Gilmore D, *et al.* (2003) Anaphylactoid syndrome of pregnancy: a review of the literature with latest management and outcome data. *AANA J.* **71**(2): 120–6.
9 Kocarev M, Lyons G. (2007) Amniotic fluid embolism. In: Dob D, Cooper G, Holdcroft A. *Crises in Childbirth: why mothers survive.* Oxford: Radcliffe Publishing.
10 Steiner P, Lushbaugh C. (1941) Maternal pulmonary embolism by amniotic fluid: as a cause of obstetric shock and unexpected deaths in obstetrics. *JAMA.* **117**(15): 1245–54.
11 Clark S, Hankins G, Dudley D, *et al.* (1995) Amniotic fluid embolism: analysis of the national registry. *Am J Obstet Gynecol.* **172**(4/1): 1158–69.
12 Tuffnell D, Johnson H. (2000) Amniotic fluid embolism: the UK register. *Hosp Med.* **61**(8): 532–4.
13 Powrie R, Levy M. (2008) Acute lung injury and acute respiratory distress syndrome. In: Rosene-Montella K, Keely E, Barbour L, *et al.*, editors. *Medical Care of the Pregnant Patient.* 2nd ed. Philadelphia: ACP Press.
14 Rogers M, Chang A. (2006) Postpartum hemorrhage and other problems of the third stage. In: James D, Steer P, Weiner C, Gonik B. *High Risk Pregnancy Management Options.* 3rd ed. Philadelphia: Elsevier.
15 Clark S. (1997) Amniotic fluid embolism: current concepts. *Contemp Rev Obstet Gynaecol.* **9**(4): 297–301.
16 Lockwood C, Bach R, Guha A, *et al.* (1991) Amniotic fluid contains tissue factor, a potent initiator of coagulation. *Am J Obstet Gynecol.* **165**(5/1): 1335–41.
17 Tuffnell D. (2007) Amniotic fluid embolism. In: Grady K, Howell C, Cox C. *Managing Obstetric Emergencies and Trauma: the Moet Course Manual.* 2nd ed. London: RCOG Press.
18 Benson M. (2007) A hypothesis regarding

complement activation and amniotic fluid embolism. *Med Hypotheses.* **68**(5): 1019–25.

19 Lewis G, editor. (2001) *Why Mothers Die 1997–1999: The fifth report of the Confidential Enquiries into Maternal Deaths in the United Kingdom.* London: RCOG Press.

20 Lawson H, Atrash H, Franks A. (1990) Fatal pulmonary embolism during legal induced abortion in the United States from 1972 to 1985. *Am J Obstet Gynecol.* **162**: 986–90.

21 Bell J, Pearn J, Wilson G, Ansford A. (1987) Prenatal cytogenetic diagnosis – a current audit. A review of 2000 cases of prenatal cytogenetic diagnoses after amniocentesis, and comparisons with early experience. *Med J Aust.* **146**: 12–15.

22 Kelly M, Bailie K, McCourt K. (1995) A case of amniotic fluid embolism in a twin pregnancy in the second trimester. *Int J Obstet Anesth.* **4**: 175–7.

23 Olcott C, Robinson A, Maxwell T, *et al.* (1973) Amniotic fluid embolism and disseminated intravascular coagulation after blunt abdominal trauma. *J Trauma.* **13**: 737–40.

24 Gilbert W, Danielsen B. (1999) Amniotic fluid embolism: decreased mortality in a population-based study. *Obstet Gynecol.* **93**: 973–7.

25 Margarson M. (1995) Delayed amniotic fluid embolism following cesarean section under spinal anaesthesia. *Anaesthesia.* **50**(9): 804–6.

26 Department of Health. (1998) *Why Mothers Die: report on confidential enquiries into maternal deaths in the United Kingdom 1994–1996.* London: The Stationery Office.

27 Benson M, Kobayashi H, Silver R, *et al.* (2001) Immunologic studies in presumed amniotic fluid embolism. *Obstet Gynecol.* **97**: 510–14.

28 Kobayashi H, Ohi H, Terao T. (1993) A simple, noninvasive, sensitive method for diagnosis of amniotic fluid embolism by monoclonal antibody TKH–2 that recognizes NeuAca2–6GaINAc. *Am J Obstet Gynecol.* **168**(3/1): 848–53.

29 Kanayma N, Yamazaki T, Naruse H, *et al.* (1992) Determining zinc coproporphyrin in maternal plasma – a new method for diagnosing amniotic fluid embolism. *Clin Chem.* **38**: 526–9.

30 Baskett T. (2004) *Essential Management of Obstetric Emergencies.* 4th ed. Bristol: Clinical Press.

31 Han D, Lee K, Franquet T, *et al.* (2003) Thrombotic and non-thrombotic pulmonary arterial embolism: spectrum of imaging findings. *Radiographics.* **23**: 1521–39.

32 Stafford I, Sheffield J. (2007) Amniotic fluid embolism. *Obstet Gynecol Clin North Am.* **34**(3): 545–53.

33 Tuffnell D. (2003) Amniotic fluid embolism. *Curr Opin Obstet Gynecol.* **15**(2): 119–22.

34 Martin R. (1996) Amniotic fluid embolism. *Clin Obstet Gynecol.* **39**(1): 101–6.

35 Moore J, Baldisseri M. (2005) Amniotic fluid embolism. *Crit Care Med.* **33**(S10): S279–85.

36 Tuffnell D, Hamilton S. (2008) Amniotic fluid embolism. *Obstet Gynaecol Reprod Med.* **18**(8): 23–26.

37 Davies S. (2001) Amniotic fluid embolus: a review of the literature. *Can J Anaesth.* **48**(1): 88–98.

38 Prosper S, Goudge C, Lupo V. (2007) Recombinant factor VIIa to successfully manage disseminated intravascular coagulation from amniotic fluid embolism. *Obstet Gynecol.* **109**(2): 524–5.

39 Gist R, Stafford I, Leibowitz A, *et al.* (2009) Amniotic fluid embolism. *Anesth Analg.* **108**(5): 1599–1602.

40 Turikllazzi E, Greco P, Neri M, *et al.* (2009) Amniotic fluid embolism: still a diagnostic enigma for obstetrician and pathologist? *Acta Obstetricia et Gynecologica Scandinavica.* **88**(7): 839–41.

41 Hayashi R. (2000) Obstetric collapse. In: Kean LH, Baker PN, Edelstone DI, editors, *Best Practice in Labour Ward Management.* Edinburgh: WB Saunders.

42 Abecassis P, Benhamou D. (2006) Is amniotic fluid embolism likely to recur in a subsequent pregnancy? *Int J Obst Anesth.* **15**: 90.

43 Demianczuk C, Corbett T. (2005) Successful pregnancy after amniotic fluid embolism: a case report. *J Obstet Gynaecol Can.* **27**(7): 699–701.

CHAPTER 12

Other causes of potential maternal collapse

Maureen Boyle

This chapter considers the less common causes of maternal conditions that need emergency or urgent attention. Note that all of these conditions fall outside the midwives' remit and therefore their role is to provide a high standard of supportive care after summoning emergency assistance or organising urgent referral.

For most of these conditions prompt medical or surgical aid is the only treatment. However, it could be that an overview of the potential causes of the woman's symptoms will help the midwife to decide how best to support her, especially in isolated situations, until assistance arrives. It is also possible that prior revision of these conditions will lead to earlier suspicion and referral of symptoms which might otherwise have progressed to an emergency situation. Knowledge of these conditions may also be useful if the midwife wishes to continue her duty of care and act as the woman's advocate.[1]

The overview given here is, of necessity, very brief and is intended to be just a summary. However, it will provide a starting point before accessing other resources for more in-depth information. Further information may also be necessary in preparation for discussing the situation with a woman who has suffered any of these conditions.

The main presenting symptoms of maternal collapse are identified in the first part of this chapter, with the conditions that may be the potential cause listed alphabetically below each one. Of course many conditions manifest with various symptoms, depending on the degree of severity or just the individual aetiology and therefore may appear in more than one list. Some of these conditions are discussed in previous chapters. Others are briefly summarised later in this chapter, presented in alphabetical order. All require urgent care.

Loss of consciousness

A useful assessment tool when evaluating level of consciousness is the Glasgow Coma Scale given in Table 12.1.

A woman with a score of less than eight on the Glasgow Coma Score is in a coma and probably needs respiratory support. If the score falls two or more points,

TABLE 12.1 The Glasgow Coma Scale

	1	2	3	4	5	6
Eyes	Does not open eyes	Opens eyes only in response to painful stimuli	Opens eyes in response to voice	Opens eyes spontaneously	N/A	N/A
Verbal	Makes no sounds	Makes sounds which cannot be understood	Uses inappropriate words	Confused, disoriented	Oriented, speaks normally	N/A
Motor	Makes no movements	Extension to painful stimuli	Abnormal flexion to painful stimuli	Flexion/ withdraws in response to painful stimuli	Can isolate painful stimuli	Obeys commands

this represents a significant deterioration in neurological condition.

A diagnosis of amniotic fluid embolism (*see* Chapter 11) should be considered at an early stage in all cases of unexplained maternal collapse.[2]

Common causes of loss of consciousness

- Acute (adult) respiratory distress syndrome (ARDS) (*see* page 182)
- Amniotic fluid embolism (*see* Chapter 11)
- Anaphylaxis (*see* page 183)
- Aneurysm: ruptured
- Asthma (*see* page 184)
- Cerebrovascular accident or stroke (*see* page 184)
- Diabetic ketoacidosis (*see* page 184)
- Drug intoxication
- Epidural: high block (*see* page 185)
- Eclampsia (*see* Chapter 4)
- Haematoma: paravaginal or paragenital (*see* page 152)
- Hyperventilation
- Hypoglycaemia (*see* page 187)

- Hypotension
- Local anaesthetic toxicity
- Magnesium toxicity (*see* Chapter 4)
- Myocardial infarction
- Peripartum cardiomyopathy (*see* page 187)
- Pulmonary embolism (*see* Chapter 3)
- Thyroid crisis (*see* page 189)
- Uterine rupture (*see* Chapter 8).

Chest pain

Because heartburn is so common a complaint in pregnancy, chest pain may not be treated with the urgency it may need in some rare cases. However, life-threatening causes usually present with severe pain, unrelieved by common medicine, and are associated with other symptoms (for example, dyspnoea, nausea, vomiting and altered consciousness). A lesson can be learned from a case in a former Report on Confidential Enquiries into Maternal Deaths[3] concerning a woman of 33 weeks' gestation who, after seeking repeat antacids from her GP (for presumably ongoing 'heartburn') and seemingly with no other signs than proteinuria and some oedema, died suddenly at home from eclampsia.

Common causes of chest pain
- Aortic dissection
- Myocardial infarction (*see* page 187)
- Pericarditis
- Peripartum cardiomyopathy (*see* page 187)
- Pleurisy
- Pneumonia
- Pneumothorax
- Pre-eclampsia: fulminating (*see* Chapter 4)
- Pulmonary embolism (*see* Chapter 3)
- Sickle-cell crisis (*see* page 188).

Confusion

Confusion may manifest not only as inappropriate speech, but also as aggression or withdrawal of communication. The midwife must make a decision on whether the cause could be a pathophysiological condition before deciding on the most appropriate action. However, it is worth noting that confusion can often be an early sign of hypoxia.

Common causes of confusion
- ARDS (*see* page 182)
- Asthma (*see* page 184)
- Cerebrovascular accident (*see* page 184)
- Drug intoxication or drug withdrawal
- Hypoglycaemia (*see* page 187)
- Hypotension
- Magnesium toxicity (*see* Chapter 4)
- Permanent mental disability
- Pre-eclampsia: fulminating (*see* Chapter 4)
- Psychiatric illness
- Pulmonary oedema (*see* page 188)

- Sepsis (*see* page 188)
- Thyroid crisis (*see* page 189).

Shock

See Chapter 2 for a full discussion on the signs, symptoms and related pathophysiology of shock.

Common causes of shock
- ARDS (*see* page 182)
- Amniotic fluid embolism (*see* Chapter 11)
- Antepartum haemorrhage (*see* Chapter 5)
- Appendicitis (*see* page 183)
- Ectopic pregnancy (*see* page 185)
- Postpartum haemorrhage (see Chapter 10)
- Pulmonary embolism (*see* Chapter 3)
- Sepsis (*see* page 188)
- Uterine inversion (*see* Chapter 8)
- Uterine rupture (*see* Chapter 8).

Abdominal pain

Abdominal pain is probably the most common presenting symptom seen by midwives, and as women manifest contraction pain in various ways, it is tempting to assume most abdominal pain is labour. However, it is worth maintaining a degree of suspicion, and considering carefully where the pain is, if there is anything that makes it worse or better, and – most importantly – whether it is intermittent, with the uterus relaxing in between.

Common causes of abdominal pain
- Antepartum haemorrhage (*see* Chapter 5)
- Appendicitis (*see* page 183)
- Ectopic pregnancy (*see* page 185)
- Fibroids (*see* page 186)

- Haematoma: rectus (*see* page 187)
- Pyelonephritis
- Renal stones (unusual in pregnancy as the renal tract is dilated)
- Thyroid crisis (*see* page 189)
- Uterine inversion (*see* Chapter 8)
- Uterine rupture (*see* Chapter 8).

Convulsion

Although the most common cause of a convulsion in pregnancy, labour or following birth is eclampsia, other more rare conditions can first present with a fit.

Common causes of convulsion
- Eclampsia (*see* Chapter 4)
- Amniotic fluid embolism (*see* Chapter 11)
- Epilepsy (*see* page 186)
- Sickle-cell crisis (*see* page 188).

Trauma

It is always possible that a midwife may be the first person on the scene following a car accident, a violent incident or other injury to a pregnant woman. In these circumstances it is possible to do no more than provide skilled first aid, remembering that the best way to care for the fetus is to adequately resuscitate the mother (*see* Chapter 2). After calling for emergency help, initial assessment and action should include the emergency measures in Box 12.1.

Other conditions
Acute (adult) respiratory distress syndrome

ARDS is usually the result of another condition (for example, amniotic fluid embolism, acute infection, eclampsia,

> **BOX 12.1** Emergency care
> **Call for help.**
> - **A**irway: maintain open. Ensure a lateral tilt or displace the uterus, while protecting the cervical and remainder of the spine.
> - **B**reathing: assist if necessary.
> - **C**irculation: control obvious bleeding if possible and give cardiac massage if necessary.
> - **D**isability: assess level of consciousness by noting response to voice or pain.
> - **E**nvironment: keep warm and safe.

abruption, aspiration or anaphylaxis) and although mortality has been quoted as high, for the survivors the long-term prognosis, even following prolonged ventilation,[4] is good with lung function recovery back to normal in four to six months in many women. However, there is also the possibility of complications as a result of ventilation and admission to an intensive therapy unit.

Women will show signs of acute respiratory distress such as tachycardia, tachypnoea and cyanosis. There will be lung crackles, and bilateral interstitial infiltrates appear on chest X-ray.[5] Diagnosis is by clinical signs, but the primary cause also needs to be diagnosed and treated concurrently.

Treatment, usually in an intensive care unit, is aimed at treating the cause and supporting lung function until the lung heals. Optimum oxygenation must be maintained and acidosis, anaemia and hypothermia prevented. Careful fluid balance is necessary to prevent pulmonary oedema, and ventilation may be necessary.

Anaphylaxis

Anaphylaxis is an acute response, with multisystem involvement, resulting from the rapid release of inflammatory mediators, to a substance to which the woman has become sensitised. The substance may commonly be a drug, food or a material such as latex. The response usually begins rapidly within seconds or minutes and a full reaction occurs within 30 minutes.

Possible signs and symptoms include urticaria, pruritis, flushing, erythema, nausea, vomiting and diarrhoea, tachycardia, laryngeal oedema, generalised oedema, bronchospasm, hypotension and respiratory or cardiac collapse.

Together with summoning urgent help, the immediate treatment is to stop any drugs and infusions, etc., administer oxygen and monitor oxygen saturations, monitor vital signs, obtain intravenous access and administer fluids to maintain blood pressure. Basic life support may be necessary (*see* Chapter 2). Blood gases must be monitored and a full blood count, electrolyte assessment and clotting studies carried out. An electrocardiograph and X-ray may be necessary. Depending on the woman's condition, a left lateral tilt may be the optimum position, and intubation and ventilation for respiratory support may be necessary.

Drug therapy is an important part of treatment and may include epinephrine, antihistamines, corticosteroids and bronchodilators.

If the woman is still pregnant, cardiotocography monitoring is appropriate and delivery may be needed, although fetal distress may be a response to maternal hypoxia and hypotension, and resolve as she is treated. The timing of delivery in these circumstances is controversial.[6] If a woman has had a suspected anaphylactic reaction, it needs investigating usually by a local allergy clinic.

Latex allergy is apparently increasing, so midwives need to suspect this cause and possibly anticipate it by asking specific questions (perhaps at booking) regarding women's previous reactions to other latex products such as condoms, balloons or household rubber gloves.[7] If latex allergy is identified, great care is needed because much midwifery equipment (such as tape, catheters, masks, etc. as well as gloves) contain latex.

Appendicitis

Appendicitis is relatively common in pregnant women, occurring in approximately 1:1500 pregnant women.[8] It is thought to be more common in the first and second trimester, but in the third trimester, perforation is more common.[9] It may be harder to diagnose in pregnancy because the gravid uterus displaces the appendix, so the pain may be higher and more lateral, although right lower quadrant pain is still the most common presenting symptom at any gestational age.[10] In addition, because of the change of position of the appendix, peritonitis is a more common complication in pregnant women.[11]

Signs and symptoms may include pain, nausea, vomiting and maybe pyrexia. Ultrasound is usually undertaken but if this is inconclusive, CT and MRI assessment may be used.[12] Treatment is surgical and necessary at any stage of pregnancy, with usually good results.[13] However, medical management may be undertaken.[14] A delay in diagnosis and treatment can lead to perforation and/ or peritonitis and potentially to maternal and fetal morbidity or mortality.[15]

Asthma

Asthma may affect up to 12% of pregnancies[16] and is the most common obstructive pulmonary disorder occurring during pregnancy.[17] The effect of pregnancy on asthma is unpredictable, but a history of asthma does seem to predispose the woman to an increased likelihood of other complications of pregnancy.[18] There is evidence that an increased severity of asthma pre-pregnancy will be reflected in an increased likelihood of problems in pregnancy.[19,20]

Signs and symptoms of an asthma attack may include increased respiration rate, increased heart rate, use of accessory muscles for breathing and bronchospasm. As the attack worsens in severity, the woman may make only a poor respiratory effort, become exhausted, cyanosed, confused and finally bradycardic and comatose. Life-threatening asthma would be considered an oxygen saturation of <92%, increasing cyanosis, hypotension and weak respiratory effort.[21]

Treatment of an asthma exacerbation includes the administration of humidified oxygen, intravenous access and fluids, drug therapy with bronchodilators or systemic steroids and ongoing assessment with pulse oximeter, ECG, X-ray, arterial blood gases, maternal peak flow and CTG if antenatal. With a severe asthma attack that is difficult to treat (status asthmaticus) and progressing to respiratory failure, intubation and ventilation are needed.

Cerebrovascular accident (CVA)

Although considered a condition of old age, strokes happen to childbearing women: one study reported an incidence of about 1:1500 pregnancies (to six weeks postnatal)[22] and with the changes in lifestyle putting increasingly younger women

at higher risk it is likely this number will rise. It has been noted that women are at increased risk of CVA in the six weeks following delivery.[22]

A stroke may be either ischaemic or haemorrhagic and symptoms are similar, although treatments will differ. An ischaemic stroke is caused by severe loss of blood flow to part of the brain; in young women, a cardioembolism is a common cause. This may be limited and cause only a transient ischaemic attack (TIA) or it may be prolonged and cause permanent damage or death. Most TIAs and about 25% of ischaemic strokes happen in the first postpartum week.[23] A haemorrhagic stroke is caused by a bleed, either intracerebral or subarachnoid, and may result from a vessel wall or other haematological abnormality.

Symptoms can range in severity from headache and mild muscle weakness to collapse and cardiac or respiratory arrest. Various investigations may be needed to determine a diagnosis, including CT scan, MRI, lumbar puncture, cerebral angiography and haematological testing.

Treatment of ischaemic stroke includes possible anticoagulation, while treatment of haemorrhagic stroke is usually surgical. Ongoing treatment needs will depend on the severity of the stroke.

Diabetic ketoacidosis

Diabetic ketoacidosis is a medical emergency affecting about 1%–3% of diabetic pregnancies and has the potential for maternal mortality.[24] However, improvement in the care of pregnant diabetic women has reduced this risk. Nevertheless, fetal mortality remains high.[24]

Diabetic ketoacidosis normally affects only those with type I diabetes, but it is not unknown in type II or even gestational diabetes.[25] A recent Confidential Enquiries into Maternal Deaths[26] included the postnatal death of a woman considered to have had gestational diabetes, so attention to follow-up care is clearly necessary. The most common cause of diabetic ketoacidosis is infection, although pyrexia may not be present.

Diabetic ketoacidosis can present as a collapse (coma) but may be preceded by excessive thirst, polyuria, abdominal pain, vomiting, hyperventilation and/or weakness. Development of ketoacidosis can be more rapid in pregnancy.[24]

Diagnosis is usually by arterial pH and a dipstick of urine may show 4+ glucose. However, in pregnancy a woman may have significant ketoacidosis with only slight serum hyperglycaemia.[28,29] Treatment includes appropriate resuscitation, then rehydration, careful blood glucose monitoring and glucose or insulin therapy as necessary. Infection must be investigated and treated. Reduced variability and decelerations on the CTG will often resolve, with improvement of the maternal condition, so caesarean section for fetal distress is not usually necessary.[30]

Ectopic pregnancy

Ectopic pregnancies are a common complication. The majority of them occur as a singleton pregnancy within the fallopian tubes. However, the occurrence of heterotopic pregnancy, a combination of ectopic and intrauterine pregnancy, is increasing and is probably due to the increase in assisted conceptions.[31]

Abdominal pain is usually felt from about four to six weeks. However, pain may be referred and it has been stated that pain anywhere from shoulder to knee in sexually active women of childbearing age should be assessed for ectopic pregnancy. Rupture and vaginal bleeding may occur from five to 10 weeks, and be accompanied by nausea and vomiting. Diagnosis is by positive pregnancy test and abdominal or vaginal ultrasound.

Treatment involves resuscitation as necessary to stabilise the woman's condition, including administering IV fluids (with blood transfusion as necessary) and laparoscopic or abdominal surgery. In an early and unruptured ectopic pregnancy, it may be possible to treat the condition medically.[32,33]

Epidural/spinal: high block

In an Australian study of 10 995 epidurals, high blocks occurred on eight occasions (0.07%) and two of these women required intubation and ventilation.[34]

High blocks may occur as a result of an unexpected spread of local anaesthetic after a subarachnoid (spinal) injection or after an accidental subarachnoid injection of an epidural dose of local anaesthetic.[35]

Signs and symptoms are dependent on the height of the block but may include tingling, weakness in hands, nausea, different breathing, hypotension and/or bradycardia. With a total spinal block, loss of consciousness will occur due to the direct action of local anaesthetic on the brain.

Immediate treatment is to turn off the epidural if running as a continuous infusion, call for urgent help and commence resuscitation if necessary. Oxygen should be given, with continuous monitoring of oxygen saturations, and frequent blood pressure readings will underpin treatment. Anaesthetists will treat hypotension and bradycardia as appropriate. The CTG will reflect the mother's condition but adequate resuscitation and treatment should maintain fetal well-being.

Epilepsy

Epilepsy is relatively common, affecting around 1:200 women attending antenatal clinics.[21] Although in general a woman with epilepsy can expect good outcomes, her pregnancy is not without risk. The Confidential Enquiries[26] have noted several deaths a year since 1988 in women with epilepsy. Many women have specific 'triggers' for their seizures (such as flashing lights or fatigue) and care should be taken to avoid these when possible.

A seizure can last for a varying amount of time. Status epilepticus is a continuous prolonged seizure lasting for 30 minutes or more, or a series of seizures (>3) when there is no recovery in between. Besides having serious potential maternal effects, this can result in premature labour, rupture of membranes, abruption or fetal death.[27]

The midwife should immediately call for urgent help and then maintain the woman's safety (e.g. ensuring she does not hit her head or fall from a bed, etc.). After the fit, the woman should be placed in the recovery position with priority being given to maintaining a patent airway. If available, oxygen should be given. If at home, transfer into hospital should be made, via ambulance. In hospital, the woman is usually cannulated and blood specimens sent as required (to include toxicology and anti-epileptic drug level). Her normal drug regime should be reviewed and changes to it may be made. If there is any question of eclampsia, magnesium sulphate will be given (see Chapter 4).

Fibroids

Fibroids are common benign tumours which can be located in the uterus. In pregnancy, they may degrade (usually causing dark red or brown vaginal loss), stay the same or grow – in which case they may compromise the growth of the fetus or cause premature labour. If they are positioned low down in the uterus, they may interfere with the lie and descent into the pelvis of the fetus, and subsequently with the mode of birth.

These conditions are not usually acute in the antenatal period, although fibroids may be a cause of postpartum haemorrhage (see Chapter 10). Rarely in pregnancy, fibroids can cause varying degrees of pain (including intolerable)[36] and this must of course be investigated, although frequently treatment is only analgesia. However if peduncular, a fibroid may twist (torsion), which could cause acute abdominal pain, vomiting and pyrexia. Diagnosis is usually by ultrasound, and surgery may be necessary.

Haematoma: paravaginal or paragenital

If a woman collapses or shows signs of shock after the third stage and there is no visible sign of haemorrhage, a concealed haemorrhage may be suspected.[37]

Although it would be expected that most severe genital tract trauma would be caused by an instrumental delivery, a past Report on Confidential Enquiries into Maternal Deaths[38] included the case of a woman giving birth to a preterm baby unattended and subsequently dying from a vaginal wall haematoma, despite treatment. There may also not be any visible trauma – a paravaginal haematoma has been reported following a spontaneous vaginal delivery with no perineal or vaginal trauma.[39]

Treatment is resuscitation as necessary, including siting an IV, and treating the cause. Depending on the site, the haematoma may be treated through the vagina or the woman may need a laparotomy.

Haematoma: rectus

This is a rare condition and occurs when a sudden spasm such as a sneeze ruptures the inferior epigastric veins and/or causes the rectus muscle to dehisce. This usually only takes place late in pregnancy when the abdominal wall is under pressure from a large uterus, but a recent report has noted an occurrence resulting in an emergency caesarean section at 30 weeks.[40]

Signs and symptoms include severe local pain and possible slight blood loss. Diagnosis is usually from symptoms, but ultrasound may be used. Treatment will depend on the severity and may be conservative or surgical.

Hypoglycaemia

Hypoglycaemia can cause rapid loss of consciousness in contrast to diabetic ketoacidosis which causes gradual loss of consciousness. It can be immediately life-threatening. Hypoglycaemia can present not only in diabetes mellitus, but also in Addison's disease, hypopituitarism and hypothyroidism. Diagnosis is by measurement of the blood glucose level.

Treatment includes resuscitation as necessary and, following assessment of blood glucose, IV administration of 50% dextrose or glucagon given intramuscularly if no IV access is possible. This should be accompanied by oxygen administration, oxygen saturation monitoring, and, if antenatal, CTG monitoring of the fetal well-being.

Myocardial infarction (MI): heart attack

MI, resulting from coronary arterial disease, is a growing problem in women of childbearing age, mainly as a result of changing lifestyles.[41] Signs and symptoms of MI include chest pain (often described as 'crushing'), pain in arms (usually left), neck, back and/or lower jaw, nausea and sweating. As initially symptoms may be mild, midwives need to keep a degree of suspicion when a woman complains of chest pain, although the cause is usually the common pregnancy ailment of heartburn. Nevertheless, careful assessment will enable midwives to appropriately refer women for diagnosis: usually by 12-lead ECG and blood tests. A severe MI is an emergency which may need immediate resuscitation and may result in treatment such as thrombolytic agents or open heart surgery. The mother is at the same risk as if she were not pregnant, but a high fetal loss has been reported.[41]

Peripartum cardiomyopathy

Peripartum cardiomyopathy is suspected when congestive cardiac failure develops in a previously fit woman towards the end of pregnancy or within about five months postnatally. Aetiology is unknown but may be a myocarditis caused by infection or an autoimmune response. The rate of maternal mortality can be about 25%–50%.

Risk factors include advanced maternal age, multiparity, twin pregnancy, long-term tocolytic therapy and perhaps cocaine abuse. Presenting signs and symptoms may include dyspnoea, tachypnoea, cough, orthopnoea, palpitations, tachycardia, haemoptysis, chest pain, abdominal pain, ascites, peripheral oedema and/or confusion.

A cardiac assessment is needed and peripartum cardiomyopathy is diagnosed after exclusion of other causes of cardiac failure. Treatment involves care by a cardiology team in a cardiac unit, with close monitoring and support of cardiac and respiratory function. If the woman is still pregnant, delivery should be expedited.

Early diagnosis is vital to ensure optimum outcome, but there may never be a full recovery.[42] If the condition persists for more than six months, it is associated with a poor outcome. There is uncertainty as to whether peripartum cardiomyopathy will recur in a future pregnancy, but studies have not generally demonstrated good outcomes.[43]

Pulmonary oedema

Pulmonary oedema is a potential complication of many conditions including pre-eclampsia, septicaemia, pulmonary embolism, amniotic fluid embolism or it may be caused by fluid overload and/or tocolytic treatment for premature labour. Fluid may enter the alveoli of the lungs due to pulmonary capillary damage or may diffuse from the vessels due to a reduction in colloid oncotic pressure.[44] This fluid will not only block effective oxygenation but also damage the alveoli.

The woman will appear breathless, tachycardic and may have haemoptysis. Diagnosis will be made on clinical signs and X-ray findings. Treatment has three aims – to maintain oxygen saturations at >95%, to treat the cause and to relieve symptoms. Respiratory support as necessary will be undertaken, drugs including diuretics in particular will be used, and careful fluid balance monitoring is vital, which may include fluid restriction. Pulmonary oedema must be effectively treated or it may progress to ARDS.

Sepsis

Although infection during or after pregnancy is a relatively common condition, it is not normally serious because childbearing women are usually young and healthy, and in the UK, infections are identified and treated. However, 18 women died of sepsis before or after delivery in a recent Report into Confidential Enquiries into Maternal Deaths[26] and although this number has been relatively unchanged for many years, it is likely to rise substantially in the future. Early signs may not always be easily recognised and fulminating septicaemia can occur rapidly.

An infected woman may be pyrexial, but this may progress to hypothermia in septic shock. Her skin may change from warm and dry to red and clammy. She will be tachycardic and confusion may be present relatively early in the process. Severe sepsis can cause organ dysfunction, hypotension despite adequate fluid intake or administration, and hypoperfusion.

Diagnosis of the source of infection is necessary. Relevant specimens (for example, urine and wound drainage) must be collected and cultured. Blood cultures should be obtained when a woman's pyrexia is at its highest, but these may not always be conclusive. A chest X-ray, ultrasound or CT scan may be appropriate but the woman may need surgery for diagnosis.

Treatment will depend on the symptoms and the woman's condition, but will involve appropriate respiratory support, antibiotics and careful monitoring of vital signs, general condition and fluid balance. She may also need surgery for drainage and/or debridement.

In the worst cases sepsis could lead to acute renal failure, respiratory failure and/or DIC, and septic shock has a mortality of 20%–50%.[45]

Sickle-cell crisis

A sickle-cell crisis is more common in pregnancy because of increased hypercoagulability, especially in the third trimester and following birth. About one-third of pregnant women with sickle-cell disease will have at least one pain crisis.[46] Care must be taken to ensure that the pain is not from a cause unrelated to the disease, for example abruption, pulmonary embolism, or fulminating pre-eclampsia. The pregnant woman with sickle-cell disease is at high risk for pre-eclampsia.[47]

Signs and symptoms will depend on the area of vaso-occlusion. Dyspnoea, chest pain, hypertension and proteinuria are all possible symptoms that may signal a sickle-cell crisis, but equally need to be investigated for the more usual pregnancy complications.

Causes may include infection, dehydration, hypotension, hypothermia, hypoxia, acidosis or venous stasis. Treatment will include the management of any pregnancy complications plus rehydration as necessary, assessment of blood results, appropriate analgesia and an infection screen. A transfusion or exchange transfusion is avoided whenever possible, but may be needed.[47]

Fetal assessment is necessary and a sickle-cell crisis may lead to an early delivery, although fetal distress during a mother's crisis often disappears as the mother is treated.

Thyroid crisis (storm)

A thyroid crisis may occur in a woman already diagnosed and treated for thyrotoxicosis (hyperthyroidism) or in a woman where the disease has not been diagnosed. It can be caused by failure to take prescribed antithyroid drugs or can be precipitated by stress following infection, trauma or diabetic ketoacidosis. In one study which reported on three maternal deaths, it was suggested that caesarean section for fetal distress was the precipitating factor in two cases,

while chest infection was responsible for the other.[48]

Signs and symptoms include extreme symptoms of hyperthyroidism, such as pyrexia, tachycardia, congestive cardiac failure, abdominal pain and/or diarrhoea, hypertension, confusion, psychosis and coma.[49] The condition would obviously be suspected more readily if the woman was already known to be diagnosed with thyrotoxicosis. It is necessary to treat the pyrexia and any infection, as well as treating any cardiac failure and administering specific thyroid therapies.

References

1 Thomas BG. (1998) The disempowering concept of risk. *Pract Midwife.* 1(12): 18–21.

2 Hayashi R. (2000) Obstetric collapse. In: Kean LH, Baker PN, Edelstone DI, editors. *Best Practice in Labour Ward Management.* London: WB Saunders.

3 Department of Health. (1998) *Why Mothers Die: report on confidential enquiries into maternal deaths in the United Kingdom 1994–1996.* London: The Stationery Office.

4 Catanzarite V, Willms D, Wong D, *et al.* (2001) Acute respiratory distress syndrome in pregnancy and the puerperium: causes, courses and outcomes. *Obstet Gynecol.* 97(5/1): 760–4.

5 Lewis P, Lanouette J. (2000) Principles of critical care. In: Cohen W, editor. *Cherry and Merkatz's Complications of Pregnancy.* 5th ed. London: Lippincott, Williams & Wilkins.

6 Chaudhuri K, Gonzales J, Jesurun C, *et al.* (2008) Anaphylactic shock in pregnancy: a case study and review of the literature. *Int J Obstet Anesth.* 17(4): 350–7.

7 Draisci G, Nucera E, Pollastrini E, *et al.* (2007) Anaphylactic reactions during cesarean section. *Int J Obstet Anesth.* 16(1): 63–7.

8 Miller M. (2008) Gastrointestinal disorders. In: Rosene-Montella K, Keely

E, Barbour L, *et al.*, editors. *Medical Care of the Pregnant Patient*. 2nd ed. Philadelphia: ACP Press.

9 Cox C. (2002) Abdominal emergencies in pregnancy. In: Grady K, Howell C, Cox C. *Managing Obstetric Emergencies and Trauma: the Moet Course Manual*. 2nd ed. London: RCOG Press.

10 Mouad J, Elliott J, Erickson L, *et al.* (2000) Appendicitis in pregnancy: new information that contradicts long-held clinical beliefs. *Am J Obstet Gynecol*. **182**(5): 1027–9.

11 Baskett T. (2004) *Essential Management of Obstetric Emergencies*. 4th ed. Bristol: Clinical Press Limited.

12 Basaran A, Basaran M. (2009) Diagnosis of acute appendicitis during pregnancy: a systematic review. *Obstet Gynecol Surv*. **64**(7): 481–8.

13 Kilpatrick C, Monga M. (2007) Approach to the acute abdomen in pregnancy. *Obstet Gynecol Clin North Am*. **34**(3): 389–402.

14 Young B, Hamar B, Levine D, *et al.* (2009) Medical management of ruptured appendicitis in pregnancy. *Obstet Gynecol*. **114**(2/2): 453–6.

15 Abbott J. (1999) Emergency management of the obstetric patient. In: Burrow G, Duffy T, editors. *Medical Complications during Pregnancy*. 5th ed. Philadelphia: WB Saunders.

16 Rey E, Boulet L. (2007) Asthma in pregnancy. *BMJ*. **334**: 582–5.

17 Bhatia P, Bhatia K. (2000) Pregnancy and the lungs. *Postgrad Med J*. **76**(901): 683–9.

18 Lui S, Wen S, Demissie K, *et al.* (2001) Maternal asthma and pregnancy outcomes: a retrospective cohort study. *Am J Obstet Gynecol*. **184**(2): 90–6.

19 Murphy V, Gibson P, Talbot P, *et al.* (2005) Severe asthma exacerbations during pregnancy. *Obstet Gynecol*. **106**(5/1): 1046–54.

20 Nelson-Piercy C. (2001) Asthma in pregnancy. *Thorax*. **56**: 325–8.

21 Nelson-Piercy C. (2006) *Handbook of Obstetric Medicine*. 3rd ed. London: Informa Healthcare.

22 Jaigobin C, Silver F. (2000) Stroke and pregnancy. *Stroke*. **31**: 2948–51.

23 Donaldson J. (1999) Neurological complications. In: Burrow G, Duffy T, editors. *Medical Complications during Pregnancy*. 5th ed. Philadelphia: WB Saunders.

24 Keely E, Montoro M. (2008) Type 1 and type 2 diabetes. In: Rosene-Montella K, Keely E, Barbour L, *et al.*, editors. *Medical Care of the Pregnant Patient*. 2nd ed. Philadelphia: ACP Press.

25 Newton C, Raskin P. (2004) Diabetic ketoacidosis in Type 1 and Type 2 diabetes mellitus: clinical and biochemical differences. *Arch Intern Med*. **164**: 1925–31.

26 Lewis G. (ed) (2007) *The Confidential Enquiry into Maternal and Child Health (CEMACH). Saving Mothers' Lives: reviewing maternal deaths to make motherhood safer 2003–2005. The Seventh Report on Confidential Enquiries into Maternal Deaths in the UK*. London: CEMACH.

27 Carhuapoma J, Tomlinson M, Levine S. (2006) Neurological disorders. In: James D, Weiner C, Steer P, *et al.*, editors. *High Risk Pregnancy: management options*. 3rd ed. Philadelphia: Elsevier Saunders.

28 Guo R, Yang L, Li L, *et al.* (2008) Diabetic ketoacidosis in pregnancy tends to occur at lower blood glucose levels: case-control study and a case report of euglycemic diabetic ketoacidosis in pregnancy. *J Obstet Gynaecol Res*. **343**(3): 324–30.

29 Chico M, Levine S, Lewis D. (2008) Normoglycemic diabetic ketoacidosis in pregnancy. *J Perinatol*. **28**(4): 310–12.

30 Richards E, Barkshire K, Russell R. (2001) Asthma, diabetic ketoacidosis and fetal distress. *Int J Obstet Anesth*. **10**(4): 317–20.

31 Jibodu O, Darne F. (1997) Spontaneous heterotopic pregnancy presenting with tubal rupture. *Hum Reprod*. **12**: 1098–9.

32 Hajenius P, Mol B, Bossuyt P, *et al.* (2001) Interventions for tubal ectopic pregnancy. *The Cochrane Library*. Issue 3. Oxford: Update Software.

33 American College of Obstetricians and Gynecologists. (2008) Medical

management of ectopic pregnancy. *Obstet Gynecol.* **111**(6): 1479–85.

34 Paech M, Godkin R, Webster S. (1998) Complications of obstetric epidural analgesia and anesthesia: a prospective analysis of 10 995 cases. *Int J Obstet Anesth.* **7**(1): 5–11.

35 Grady K, Elton J. (2007) Anaesthetic complication in obstetrics. In: Grady K, Howell C, Cox C. *Managing Obstetric Emergencies and Trauma: the MOET Course Manual.* 2nd ed. London: RCOG Press.

36 Henshaw A. (2006) Uterine fibroids: potential complications and impact on pregnancy. *Br J Midwif.* **14**(2): 73–5.

37 Cox C. (2007) Abdominal emergencies in pregnancy. In: Grady K, Howell C, Cox C. *Managing Obstetric Emergencies and Trauma: the MOET Course Manual.* 2nd ed. London: RCOG Press.

38 Lewis G, editor. (2001) *Why Mothers Die 1997–1999: the fifth report of the confidential enquiries into maternal deaths in the United Kingdom.* London: RCOG Press.

39 Singh J, Basu S, Aich A, *et al.* (2008) Spontaneous ischiorectal and retroperitoneal haematoma after normal vaginal delivery. *J Obstet Gynaecol.* **28**(8): 798–9.

40 Kundodyiwa T, Thomas A, Nwosu E. (2008) A case of spontaneous rectus sheath haematoma in pregnancy. *J Obstet Gynaecol.* **28**: 795–6.

41 Roos-Hesselink J. (2006) Ischaemic heart disease. In: James D, Weiner C, Steer P, *et al.*, editors. *High Risk Pregnancy: management options.* 3rd ed. Philadelphia: Elsevier Saunders.

42 Dorbala S, Brozena S, Seb S, *et al.* (2005) Risk stratification of women with peripartum cardiomyopathy at initial presentation: a dobutamine stress echocardiography study. *J Am Soc Echocardiogr.* **18**: 45–8.

43 Elkayam U, Tummala P, Rao K, *et al.* (2001) Maternal and fetal outcomes of subsequent pregnancies in women with peripartum cardiomyopathy. *N Engl J Med.* **344**(21): 1567–71.

44 Meller J, Goldman M. (2000) Cardiopulmonary disorders. In: Cohen W, editor. *Cherry and Merkatz's Complications of Pregnancy.* 5th ed. London: Lippincott, Williams & Wilkins.

45 Vincent J, de Carvalho F, De Backer D. (2002) Management of septic shock. *Ann Med.* **34**(7–8): 606–13.

46 Khare M, Bewley S. (2004) Management of pregnancy in sickle cell disease. In: Okpala I, editor. *Practical Management of Haemoglobinopathies.* London: Blackwell.

47 Hassell K. (2008) Hemoglobinopathies and thalassemias. In: Rosene-Montella K, Keely E, Barbour L, *et al.*, editors. *Medical Care of the Pregnant Patient.* 2nd ed. Philadelphia: ACP Press.

48 Kriplani A, Buckshee K, Bhargava V, *et al.* (1994) Maternal and perinatal outcome in thyrotoxicosis complicating pregnancy. *Eur J Obstet Gynecol Reprod Biol.* **54**(3): 159–63.

49 Kenyon A, Nelson-Piercy C. (2005) Thyroid disease. In: James D, Weiner C, Steer P, *et al.*, editors. *High Risk Pregnancy: management options.* 3rd ed. Philadelphia: Elsevier Saunders.

CHAPTER 13

Psychological considerations for 'emergencies around childbirth'

Elisabeth Hallewell

This chapter considers:

- Psychological health and childbirth; an overview
- Antenatal pre-existing psychological factors
- The psychological impact of a traumatic birth
- Childbirth risk factors for post-traumatic stress
- Postnatal support and care following a birth emergency.

Introduction

Psychological care of the woman and her birth partner during a birth emergency is an important element of the management of a birth emergency. The previous chapters have focused on life-saving measures and professional considerations. The physical well-being of the woman and her baby, and professional competence, are paramount. The psychological well-being of the woman and her partner may not seem so crucial at the time of the birth emergency but can have long-lasting adverse effects. In the research undertaken by Mapp and Hudson[1] a woman

is quoted to have said: '. . . *they do what is easiest to save your life but the care of the mind is not looked at, at all*'. Also there has been concern that the use of mannequins for emergency skills training has little consideration of the patient's viewpoint.[1]

Postnatal depression (PND) and postnatal/post-traumatic stress disorder (PTSD) have been shown to be more common in women following a difficult birth such as emergency caesarean section (EmCS) or operative vaginal birth[2,3] (*see* Box 13.1 for definitions). Birth trauma can also result in PTSD in fathers.[4] Depression and postnatal/post-traumatic stress (PTS) have been shown to co-occur and a pre-existing depression to increase susceptibility to PTS following a traumatic event.[5,6] The two disorders share some features, including diminished interest, feelings of detachment, and difficulties with sleep and concentration.[7] Awareness of these psychological disorders occurring should be used to inform postnatal psychological care following a birth emergency/traumatic birth. It is important to try to avoid postnatal adverse psychological sequelae; this may be assisted by being cognisant of the risk components.

BOX 13.1 Definitions

- **Postnatal depression** refers to depression identified by the Edinburgh Postnatal Depression Scale[8] or a modified version of the Beck Depression Inventory[9] to take into account ante/postnatal factors.

- **Postnatal/post-traumatic stress (PTS)** refers to symptoms of postnatal distress where all the criteria for postnatal stress disorder may not have been measured or met. Only a small percentage of women are likely to experience all the criteria.

- **Postnatal/post-traumatic stress disorder (PTSD)** refers to the disorder reflecting the criteria in the American Psychiatric Association *Diagnostic and Statistical Manual of Mental Disorders*, 4th edition.[7]

It should be noted that PTS and PTSD are used somewhat interchangeably as is the case in the literature and research.

During a birth emergency, factors shown to benefit psychological well-being and recovery following a traumatic birth should be implemented as part of the emergency management. Midwives should also take into account the body of evidence showing there is a relationship between antenatal and postnatal psychological well-being.[10] This clearly shows that psychological care needs to be addressed by those providing maternity care commencing from the first antenatal appointment, and be continued throughout the whole childbirth experience. Failure to address the woman's psychological well-being during labour and a birth emergency could have long-term ramifications for the woman and her family. White *et al.*[6] suggest that symptoms of PTSD can persist as long as 40 years after the event.

The main aim of this chapter is to equip midwives with the knowledge of factors that have been shown by research to promote the psychological well-being of the woman and her partner, when during the birth of their baby there has been an emergency. It is hoped that by implementing the recommendations indicated by research findings that women and their partners will be better assisted in coping with a traumatic birth and be able to enjoy parenthood. In addition psychological disorders associated with childbirth are discussed to enhance midwives' knowledge.

Psychological health and childbirth: an overview

Early descriptions of psychological disturbances following childbirth were associated with physical problems. Hippocrates, in his description of 'milk fever', mentioned symptoms of weeping and hysteria.[11] Louis-Victor Marcé (1828–64), a Parisian physician, was one of the first in recognising the existence of mental distress specifically relating to childbirth,[12] but toxaemia and sepsis were common causes of puerperal psychoses around this time. Also fears of complications of childbirth in the 19th century and early 20th century led to maternal apprehension and depression. Shorter, in his chapter on pain and death in childbirth, includes a quote from a working-class woman around 1914, 'I always prepared myself to die, and I think this awful depression is common to most at this time.'[13] Recognition in the 1930s that women may have psychological problems associated with childbirth and lactation was acknowledged by the Infanticide Act 1932. This act considered that a woman who was responsible for the death of her baby (up to one year) could be considered to have committed infanticide, rather than murder, as a result of her mind being disturbed. Altered mental states following childbirth were largely thought to be a result of the reproductive process; women were at the mercy of their problematic biology. Oakley[14] suggests menstruation and childbirth are beyond the understanding of men and this resulted in medical psychiatric diagnoses of premenstrual tension and PND. Thus, unhappiness after childbirth, frequently a result of a defective social structure,[14] became more or less universally labelled as PND, which was considered a result of defective psychology of individuals affected. Postnatal mental health needs to be considered in the social context rather than being seen as an individual's psychological or biological problem, as may be the case in a biomedical approach, where 'the women's feelings are reduced to a matter of hormonal imbalance'.[15] The positive effect of social support has been shown in studies of postnatal well-being.[16,17]

The two psychological problems associated with childbirth are PND and PTSD. Mild and moderate PND has been considered largely to have its roots in the biophysical and psychosocial domains and has been accepted as a postnatal illness since 1968, when it was described by a psychiatrist called Pitt.[18,19] PND is relatively common with an incidence of 8%–15%;[19] when it is transient, lasting no longer than a few days following childbirth, it is referred to as postpartum (or 'baby') blues. If it lasts beyond a week and results in impairment in the woman's ability to function it is known as PND. Puerperal psychosis is often considered with PND, but it is much more severe and rare, affecting about 1:1000 new mothers.[19] Unlike depression, it is a psychotic disorder involving delusions, hallucinations and gross impairment in functioning, usually requiring inpatient treatment.[20] Postnatal depression may also occur in fathers. This is discussed by Beck and Driscoll[21] and the incidence of postpartum depressive symptoms in fathers is estimated to be 10%–28%. The onset of postpartum depression appears to occur later in the postpartum period in fathers, and studies have shown it to be significantly correlated to postpartum depression in their partner/spouse.[21]

Unlike PND, PTSD has not been accepted to be a result of childbirth until more recently. This in part seems to be because the symptoms associated with PTSD in men, when seen in women, were interpreted differently. Women having these symptoms were at risk of being labelled emotional and/or neurotic; alternatively, the symptoms were seen as an adjunct to PND. This is discussed later when the evidence that PTSD can occur as a result of childbirth is examined. Another issue was the Diagnostic and Statistical Manual of Mental Disorders (DSM) diagnosis and criteria for PTSD; prior to 1994 this was more restricted and could less easily be applied to birth trauma.

PTSD was outlined following the First and Second World Wars, it was often described as 'shell shock' and the description of it in DSM-I (1952) and II (1968) was of reactions to traumatic events that were seen as temporary and having an endogenous aetiology.[22] As knowledge of the disorder increased the diagnosis and criteria for PTSD included more stressors and a more general picture of post-trauma anxiety appeared.[22] This meant that in DSM-III[23] the stressors extended more widely from military combat to include stressors such as rape, but there was still controversy about the stressors that could lead to a diagnosis of PTSD. The diagnostic criteria were restricted to events 'outside the range of usual human experience',[23] and childbirth did not fit comfortably with this. Even with further modifications in DSM-IV, which take into account that PTSD may occur in individuals who are not exposed to an unusual event or even to an acute stressor,[7] controversy continues. However, this change was an important one in that it recognised that an individual's perception of a threat and response to an event can affect the subsequent development of PTSD. The broadening of the diagnostic criteria has enabled consideration of PTSD as a consequence of childbirth by researchers and clinicians[24] (*see* Box 13.2 for diagnostic criteria).

BOX 13.2 DSM-IV diagnostic criteria for PTSD as applied to childbirth[7]

A The person has been exposed to a traumatic event, i.e. childbirth, which involved threatened or actual death, or serious injury, or a threat to the physical integrity of the woman or her baby. The woman or partner's response involved intense fear, helplessness or horror.

B The traumatic birth is persistently re-experienced; the ways this may occur includes: recurrent distressing recollections of the birth, recurrent nightmares of dying or the baby dying, flashbacks, and distress on exposure to cues such as sexual intercourse and anniversary of the birth.

C Persistent avoidance of stimuli relating to the birth and including three of the following: efforts to avoid thoughts, feelings and conversations associated with the trauma, efforts to avoid things that arouse recollections of the trauma, inability to recall an important aspect of the trauma, marked diminished responsiveness in significant activities, feeling of detachment from others, restricted range of feelings, sense of foreshortened future.

D Persistent symptoms of increased arousal indicated by at least two of the following: difficulty in falling or staying asleep, irritability or outbursts of anger, difficulty concentrating, hypervigilance (of baby), exaggerated startle response.

E Duration of criteria B, C and D is more than one month.

F The disturbance causes significant distress or impairment in social, occupational or other areas of functioning.

PTSD is described as *acute* if symptoms are present for less than three months, *chronic* if the symptoms persist for three months or more and *delayed* if the onset of symptoms is at least six months after the stressor.

Ideas relating to the psychological sequelae of childbirth have moved from the perception that any problems were endogenous, being a result of the woman's biology, to being largely a result of outside factors, which can be mediated to improve women's postnatal psychological well-being. Thus midwives have a key mediation role to help to facilitate an environment that promotes women's mental health in childbirth. In order to do this, midwives also need to consider that the psychological effects of childbirth, as with any psychological response, are affected by numerous variables. Those relating to childbirth include:

- the psychological type or personality of the individual
- previous life experiences and mental health
- social support available
- expectations of birth and becoming a parent
- antenatal well-being
- the birth experience
- postnatal well-being and experience.

These variables interact, with the result that women and their partners will respond differently to experiences the midwife may feel are similar. For example, Ryding et al[25] in their study of 25 women's experiences of EmCS found that positive expectations turning into disappointment resulted in the highest prevalence (two-thirds of the women) of post-traumatic intrusive stress reactions six weeks after the birth. In this study women identified as 'confident whatever happened' had no signs of PTS whereas women who had fears that came true all perceived the birth as traumatic and a third had signs of PTS.

For the midwife to try to understand why women respond differently, risk factors for PTS and depression after birth need to be explored. The factors suggested above may provide some clues and will be considered further. These factors relate to what has happened before the pregnancy and what happens during the pregnancy and childbirth, thus providing a holistic view.

Antenatal pre-existing psychological factors

Pre-existing factors, which have been found to increase the risk of PTSD following childbirth, include:[5]

- depression in (early) pregnancy
- fear of childbirth (severe)
- pre-traumatic stress
- low stress coping (low self-esteem and self-efficacy)
- previous psychological problems
- history of psychological counselling related to childbirth
- vulnerable women.

Previous psychosocial problems, such as domestic violence and sexual abuse, are examples of factors that result in women being more vulnerable to further psychological problems. In a study undertaken by Menage[26] almost a third of women found to have diagnostic criteria for PTSD following obstetric and/or gynaecological experiences gave a prior history of sexual abuse or rape. There is also a suggestion that people have different thresholds for trauma in the same way as people are thought to have for pain.[27] This may partly explain why women who appear similar respond differently to what appear to be similar situations. Midwives caring for women during birth emergencies will need to be aware that by providing evidence-based psychological care they may be able to reduce the incidence of adverse psychological sequelae, but not eliminate it, due to the severity of the birth emergency, the woman's psychosocial background and the woman's threshold for trauma.

The importance of identifying mental health and psychosocial factors has been recognised as a key issue following findings of maternal mortality reports,[28] which have shown that suicide is a leading cause of maternal death (although suicide rates are similar to the general female population). These findings have indicated that more attention needs to be paid to mental health issues when providing maternity care. Between 2003 and 2005, 37 women committed suicide; these deaths provide an indication to the prevalence of mental distress. Seven of the deaths were attributed to severe depressive illness and three to anxiety/depressive adjustment. Thus, depression and PTSD (which is described as an anxiety disorder) are shown to be risk factors. If mental health problems are identified antenatally, informed efforts could be made to provide appropriate care throughout the maternity experience, and potentially improve psychological well-being should a birth emergency occur.

In the 2007 CEMACH report, a reduction in the number of suicides was noted and attributed to better care following recommendations from the previous report.[28] These recommendations are reflected in NICE guidelines[10] that provide guidance for the prediction, detection and initial management of metal health issues, and for preventing mental disorders. They recommend routine enquiry (*see* Box 13.3) to identify women who have or may be at risk of mental health problems.[10] With regards to preventing

mental health problems they recommend treatment of sub-threshold symptoms in pregnant women and support following traumatic birth and stillbirth. These guidelines are reinforced by CEMACH[28] where it is recommended that midwives check on the mental health of their clients twice during pregnancy and following birth.

BOX 13.3 NICE recommendations[10]

At a woman's first contact with primary care, at her booking visit and postnatally (usually at four to six weeks and three to four months), healthcare professionals (including midwives, obstetricians, health visitors and GPs) should ask two questions to identify possible depression.

- During the past month, have you often been bothered by feeling down, depressed or hopeless?
- During the past month, have you often been bothered by having little interest or pleasure in doing things?

A third question should be considered if the woman answers 'yes' to either of the initial questions.

- Is this something you feel you need or want help with?

The issues of mental illness and pre-existing psychosocial problems are largely beyond the scope of this chapter except where they have a direct impact on the woman's ability to cope with a traumatic birth. Women with a mental health illness require specialist care. However, the principles of effective psychological care may be applied to all women and their partners. If women do have depression or PTSD following a previous traumatic birth and this has not been addressed it may have an adverse effect on any subsequent pregnancy. Midwives therefore need to be aware of care that supports women following a birth emergency as well as being aware of how to promote antenatal psychological well-being.

Pre-traumatic stress, general anxiety and fear of childbirth have been shown to be the factors most strongly related to PTS and depression a month after the birth.[2,5] These antenatal factors in some cases as indicated above may be related to previous births. Zar *et al*,[29] in a study of anxiety disorder and fear of childbirth in late pregnancy, found all six multiparous women with PTSD in their study had a previous birth as the traumatic event. These women had a phobic fear of childbirth, and identification of this symptom of PTSD may not happen until a subsequent pregnancy when the woman expresses her fear of childbirth. As well as having a negative impact on subsequent pregnancies,[22] fear of childbirth has also been shown to cause some women to avoid having subsequent children.[30] The impact of unresolved PTSD is therefore profound.

The psychological impact of a traumatic birth

The woman's perception of her birth being traumatic could be expected to lead to negative psychological repercussions. However, perceptions and the ability to deal with traumatic experiences are affected by the variables identified earlier. Midwives always need to be mindful that their perception of what constitutes a traumatic birth may be different from the woman's interpretation of her experience. By monitoring this and by

avoiding factors that have been identified as contributing to women's psychological problems midwives can make a positive contribution to the psychological well-being of the women they provide care for. Providing care that promotes a positive birth experience has been highlighted in government policy for maternity care.[31-33] These reports all state that midwives and others providing care should work in partnership with women. Sadly, literature and research into PTSD indicates that some cases of PTSD may be wholly or partially as a result of these government policies not being followed. The experience of undergoing a birth emergency could be expected to be traumatic for a woman and as such will create challenges for the team providing care to promote a positive experience. They will feel their priorities are to the physical well-being of the mother and baby, but a bit more consideration of the mother as a person may make a big difference to her and her partner.

Awareness of women's traumatic experiences of childbirth, and the resulting psychological problems, increased when campaigners from organisations such as the Association for Improvement of Maternity Services (AIMS) and National Childbirth Trust (NCT) spoke and wrote of women's experiences. An example of this is a letter written in 1985 by Beech and Robinson to the Editor of the *British Journal of Psychiatry*[34] concerning women suffering 'severe nightmares' a year or more following childbirth. The term PTSD was not used, but the symptom of 'severe nightmares' is one associated with PTSD. They also identified mediating factors including 'excessively painful and traumatic deliveries', 'unsympathetic staff', experience of 'technological rape' and the 'impossibility to discuss criticism of previous care'. Several authors including Kitzinger[35,36] describe quality of care factors, such as poor communication and lack of control over what was happening, causing subsequent distress. She provides graphic examples by using quotes from women: 'They didn't speak to me. Only about me.',[35] 'felt like an oven-trussed turkey'.[35] Poor communication and lack of control are described as key issues leading to PTS after childbirth.

A study of 825 women's experiences of childbirth undertaken by Green, Coupland and Kitzinger[37] explored women's expectations and identified both positive and negative experiences. The issues they identified affecting women's overall satisfaction with birth included their feelings about major/minor interventions, pain and pain relief, control, relationship with the staff, amount and accuracy of information, and ability to get into a comfortable position. When assessing 'emotional well-being' following birth a relationship was found between having or not having interventions. This was not so much to do with whether they had the intervention or not but the context in which the decision was made. The woman's perception of the 'rightness' of the intervention was seen to be more important for her emotional well-being than the intervention itself. Women who felt the right decision had been made were significantly happier; this again reflects the importance of good communication and involvement of women with their care.

With regards to PTSD following a woman's traumatic experience of childbirth a body of psychological research has provided further information and evidence. This all should increase knowledge and understanding.

Lyons,[38] when writing about PTSD following childbirth, cites evidence from numerous studies. Several of the studies referred to compare a traumatic birth experience as being similar to a sexual assault. She concludes by suggesting that the incidence of women experiencing PTS at a level that is 'distressing and disruptive' could be shown to be greater by further studies on the incidence.[38]

The incidence of PTSD and PTS as a result of childbirth varies in the studies depending on the methods used and whether all the DSM–IV criteria are met; rates between 1% and 7% are described by Soderquist et al.[39] The number of women identifying their birth as a traumatic event is much higher than this, at around 33%,[40] but the majority of these women do not develop PTSD. The prevalence of a PTSD profile appears to be fairly stable over the first year, leading researchers to conclude women with PTSD do not all recover spontaneously.[6,39] Although studies show some variation in research methods and findings, they consistently indicate that PTSD can occur as a result of childbirth and that it may not resolve spontaneously. However, there is some evidence that a larger proportion of women do spontaneously recover from postnatal PTSD compared with women experiencing PTSD after other traumatic events such as rape.[41]

PTSD may also occur in fathers witnessing a traumatic birth involving their partner and/or baby.[4,42] In Western society there is an expectation by partners, friends and family that the father attends the birth of his children and while the majority of fathers do this willingly some are ambivalent and nervous. For some fathers being present at the birth can be 'distressing and distasteful'[43] even if there are no complications. The study by Ayers et al.[42] showed that 5% of men and women had severe symptoms of PTSD; other studies have shown rates for men to be approximately half that for women.[44-46] The symptoms were found to be strongly associated within couples, and related to similar birth factors.

The study undertaken by White[4] investigated the experience of fathers witnessing a traumatic birth. A purposive sample of 21 fathers, who provided their birth stories, was recruited through the Trauma and Birth Support group website (www.tabs.org.nz). All the participants had been distressed by their experience and had bad memories, although not all described symptoms of PTSD. Quotes included: 'Our birthing experience was a traumatic one', 'my single worst experience', 'Took three days to get over the scene, shock, did not take it in I was a dad . . . I can describe everything in the room, smells, sounds, colours. I can still see the images . . . causes headaches . . . clinical smells get you going. I resigned from my hospital laboratory job.'[4] These findings clearly show that fathers can experience similar negative psychological outcomes as mothers following a traumatic birth.

In addition to PTSD the incidence of PND may also increase as a result of a traumatic birth. However, the strongest predictor for PND is identified as antenatal depression.[47] PND has been reported to be present in a significant number of women with PTSD after childbirth.[5,6,24,39,48,49] This has also been shown to be the case with fathers.[44] The consistent findings of a high comorbidity of PND and PTSD appear to be associated with risk factors the two conditions share and that a pre-existing depression increases the risk of PTSD.[5] It is important that the

diagnosis is correct for appropriate treatment to be provided. White et al.[6] suggest that if there is a high degree of overlap between PND and PTSD, PTSD may be missed. They cite cases of women who experienced a traumatic birth and subsequently experience upsetting thoughts, being diagnosed with PND by their general practitioners. Joseph and Bailham[50] point out that only routine screening for PND can mean that PTSD is missed and that the treatment for these two conditions is different. Drug treatments may help PND, but psychological therapies are thought to be more appropriate for PTSD.

Childbirth risk factors for PTSD

As identified earlier, it is the woman's perception of childbirth, and the support she received, that are important for her psychological well-being. Midwives and others who provide care need to acknowledge that their perception of what happened may not be the same as the woman or her partner's perception. Beck[51] described a traumatic birth as being 'in the eye of the beholder'. This was the conclusion she came to after investigating 40 women's experiences of traumatic births. From the women's descriptions of their births Beck identified four main themes: these related to care, communication, trust and price of the outcome. She also listed the birth traumas identified by the 40 women in her sample.[51] The traumas she identified are largely similar to those identified in other studies (*see* Box 13.4 for summary of potential birth traumas).

The women's experiences of birth trauma include aspects of childbirth that may not have been recognised by midwives and other carers, for example

---

BOX 13.4 Summary of potential birth traumas

- Inadequate medical care/felt that staff did not know what they were doing
- Degrading experience/unsympathetic staff
- Fear of epidural/felt coerced into having an epidural
- Inadequate pain relief
- Severe pre-eclampsia/eclampsia
- Prolonged, painful labour
- Premature birth
- Emergency caesarean section/fetal distress/fear for baby's life
- Forceps/vacuum extraction
- Rapid delivery
- Postpartum haemorrhage/manual removal of placenta
- Fear for own life (maternal collapse/cardiac arrest)
- Separation from infant in neonatal intensive care unit
- Stillbirth/infant death.

'inadequate medical care' and 'degrading experience'. Ayers *et al.*[42] point out that research shows that subjective factors such as perceived support and control may be more important than objective factors such as type of delivery for the development of postnatal PTSD.

Subjective factors, as well as having a negative impact, may also alleviate the effects of a complicated birth. In a study[52] of the effects of EmCS a woman was quoted concerning her experience of a second EmCS:

'I really feel as though I was given every possible chance to achieve what I wanted. Nobody forced anything on me. I can only look back positively. Even though I ended up with an emergency caesarean section it was absolutely the right decision.'[52]

Creedy *et al.*[40] also found that women experiencing a high level of obstetric intervention were less likely to develop PTSD if they perceived their intrapartum care to have been adequate.

However, as previously indicated, the incidence of PTSD has been shown to be higher where birth complications/interventions have occurred. Many of the birth traumas listed in Box 13.4 are associated with emergencies around childbirth, for example severe pre-eclampsia/eclampsia, EmCS, forceps/vacuum delivery, premature birth, separation from baby, haemorrhage, and maternal collapse/cardiac arrest. The majority of psychological research focuses on the prevalence of PTSD and the factors that are associated with it. Although this provides valuable information, the detail that may assist midwives and other carers is not always provided. A study that does provide detail in respect to obstetric emergencies is one undertaken by two research midwives.[1] They undertook a study of 10 women's experiences of obstetric emergencies that included cord prolapse, placental abruption, shoulder dystocia, uterine scar rupture, severe pre-eclampsia, and major obstetric haemorrhage. The interviews they undertook highlight practice issues that need to be considered to improve the woman's experience and recollection of the event.

The findings of Mapp and Hudson[1] are directly related to emergencies around childbirth and are discussed in more detail than other studies for this reason. The significant themes they identify include communication and the need to make sense of what had happened. With regards to communication the women were very aware of non-verbal cues such as fear being expressed in the facial expression of the healthcare professionals. The women were therefore aware that something was wrong without being told, and were frightened when they did not know what was happening. They also commented on being reassured by receiving a smile. Touch was also identified as being important as it made the woman feel she was a human being. This contrasted with staff communicating with each other and ignoring the woman.

Information given during an emergency situation, although appreciated, may not be understood and explanations may be required later. A mother illustrates this in a study undertaken by Calam *et al.*[53] She said:

'I had fulminating toxaemia. They took the trouble to explain everything. What they'd do, how they'd make the incision. Another doctor explained about premature babies and their chances. I felt supported. Even the anaesthetist bothered to see me. I was a person.'

Did you understand?

'No. I was too upset and involved.'[53]

The women in Mapp and Hudson's[1] study appreciated that the staff were probably shocked by the situation too, and needed to manage the emergency. They provided a variety of experiences; positives included anaesthetists and midwives providing explanations and support. There were comments with regards to communication with their partners, with instances of the woman thinking there was a problem relating to them when their partner was called aside to change out of theatre clothing. The positioning of the partner in theatre and 'the green sheet' impaired communication. They felt disorientated and restricted in theatre. The women recalled experiences such as staff running down a corridor and the air blowing on their face, inexplicable pain, drifting off and then feeling better when blood transfusions were up. In most cases the women felt the situation was in the medical domain and recognised they did not have the knowledge to influence the management or outcome.

The women felt fearful for their baby's mortality but appeared to trust the healthcare professionals would help them, despite lack of explanations. They viewed continuity of carers and familiar faces positively, and felt secure when staff showed concern. However, there were instances described where the women did not feel listened to and false reassurances did not validate their situation and how they felt. The women were concerned that their partners were looked after and kept informed. They looked to their partners for support, such as holding their hand and reassurance, but recognised that they would be frightened too.

Further suggestions for midwives and other birth attendants are identified in research undertaken by Ayers.[54] Ayers' study aimed to explore issues that might be important in the development of PTS. It compared women with and without PTS following similar birth experiences. The sample had a high incidence of birth complications, due to this being the case for women with PTS, and those without PTS being matched. Twenty-five women in each group were interviewed three months after giving birth about their experiences, to examine their thoughts and emotions during birth, and their subsequent cognitive processing. Some themes identified from the interviews were common, for example poor understanding and feeling scared. Those with PTS felt more panic-y, helpless, angry and discouraged, and had more thoughts of death, mental defeat and dissociation. The thoughts of death were not always in response to a life-threatening situation showing that women can fear death without a medical reason or trigger. Midwives and other carers need to be sensitive to women's fears and reassure women and their partners by appropriately preventing or minimising the perception of life threat. The theme of anger may relate to not being listened to and not being happy about the care given. However, in some cases it may be due to the birth not going to plan despite the best efforts of the birth attendants. Anger appears to exacerbate and perpetuate PTS symptoms. Steps should be taken to recognise negative emotions to avoid mental defeat and dissociation, and when negative emotions are evident the woman should be supported as much as possible.

The experiences of fathers during birth emergencies have largely been neglected, with the focus being on the woman and her baby. The themes identified as encapsulating fathers' traumatic experiences in White's[4] study related to being a spectator, not being included, feeling sexually scarred and having to 'tough it out'. Fathers are under pressure to witness the birth of their baby, but their role is not always clear. They are expected to be a support, a fetcher and carrier, and a spectator but not necessarily a participant. They felt alienated, excluded and disregarded. The following quotes from the study illustrate these feelings:

'felt like an appendage in the way', 'not being given any information', 'I was rushed to the corner of the delivery suite and told not to interfere . . . it's like you don't count', 'evidence of midwife only working with the mother'.[4] These quotes clearly indicate that they were not being given information and support. Lack of support is further shown in the theme 'toughing it out', where fathers describe being fearful of losing their partner and unborn child, and coping by breaking down in private. They felt disempowered and unable to help their partner.

The fathers in the study were all keen to be involved, but the pressure to witness led a few to experience sexual scarring, affecting their ability to resume a sexual relationship with their partner. Three fathers declared never to have any more children. A survey of 140 fathers in New Zealand found that 100% valued a separate 'dads' group' during the antenatal course and to be able to talk with 'dads' who had 'been there, done that' to prepare them for the birth.[55] Antenatal preparation could be expected to assist both pregnant women and their partners in coping with a traumatic birth and avoid them being *totally unprepared*.[4] Several feelings such as being scared, fearful, helpless and angry were common to mothers and fathers[4,54] experiencing PTS. Both mothers and fathers have shown awareness and concern about the support given to partners during a birth emergency. A woman in Mapp and Hudson's[1] study commented, 'He had a midwife with him making sure he was kept up to date.' This would, of course, be ideal practice.

It is important that psychological care during childbirth is provided for both the woman and her partner. Fathers, as well as mothers, need to be psychologically supported for good postnatal outcomes. All the men in White's[4] study experienced subsequent marital difficulties. If midwives focus exclusively on 'being with woman' the outcome will not be optimal for the couple. Sociocultural factors are not discussed in the literature and research, but where a language barrier impairs communication it is very likely that this will have a negative impact on the already traumatic experience of a birth emergency. For these women and their partners non-verbal communication and continuity of carer will be important strategies to reduce the emotional trauma of the situation. Interpreters should be used where possible (*see* Box 13.5 for strategies to minimise emotional trauma during a birth emergency).

BOX 13.5 Midwifery strategies to minimise emotional trauma during a birth emergency

- Communicate with the woman and her partner. If the doctors do not communicate directly, convey what they are saying to the woman and her partner.
- Provide simple explanations of what is happening.
- Listen and respond to anything the woman and/or her partner say.
- Ensure adequate pain relief.
- Avoid false reassurance.
- Avoid inappropriate comments, e.g. suggesting the baby is causing problems to the parents.

- Use touch to support the woman.
- Position partner to enable easy communication with the woman where possible.
- Positively acknowledge any support the partner provides.
- Be aware of facial expressions; try to show encouragement and that you care.
- Try to provide continuity of carer.
- Introduce staff to the woman and her partner.

Postnatal support and care following a birth emergency

Following a birth emergency, where possible and appropriate, skin to skin contact with the newborn baby and an early breastfeed should be encouraged and facilitated to promote parental infant attachment, newborn thermoregulation and successful breast feeding.[56] Breast feeding has been shown to empower the new mother and benefit mental as well as physical health in women choosing to breastfeed.[57] It is therefore particularly important that women experiencing a birth emergency should receive all the support they need to enable them to breastfeed their babies. If the mother is unwell, skin to skin contact may be with the father if desired.[58] Parents with infants requiring intensive or special care will require additional support to promote parental bonding and cope with anxieties regarding the well-being of their baby.[59–61] Ayers *et al.*[42] state that it has been proposed that PTSD may impair the mother–infant bond, with symptoms either of avoiding the baby or overvigilance. Their study of 64 couples, of which 5% had PTSD symptoms, did not show that PTSD symptoms were associated with the couple's relationship or parent–baby bond. As Ayers *et al.*[42] acknowledge, their study was small and other research has shown that postnatal psychopathology is associated with poor mother–infant attachment[62] and marital relationship.[63] There is some evidence that postnatal depression can have a negative impact on mother–infant bond. Beck and Driscoll[21] and Green *et al.*[37] found that women's descriptions of their babies were more negative if they had poor 'emotional well-being' postnatally.

Mapp[64] analysed women's feelings following a birth emergency using evidence from the 10 women interviewed for a study of their feelings and fears during a birth emergency.[1] The women felt 'shell shocked' and emotional, they experienced nightmares and were frightened to be alone in the initial postnatal period. They were unable to process what had happened to them and lacked understanding of why the emergency had happened. This lack of understanding led two of the women not to be aware of how ill they had been and take appropriate care of their health postpartum. In the initial postnatal period the women had 'felt in a fog' and were unsure of the amount of information they would have been able to take in. This highlights the necessity for the midwife to be available to answer questions at a time appropriate to the individual woman.

Postnatal factors such as additional stress, support and the meanings attached to birth events may influence the development of PTSD.[41] Postnatal support should include the care recommended in NICE guidelines for postnatal care and respond to individual needs[65] to avoid any additional stress. For example, women experiencing a birth emergency may have had interventions resulting in postnatal pain; therefore, midwives need to ensure analgesia is provided and effective. The experience of postnatal pain can be overwhelming and it has been shown to contribute to PTS symptoms.[40] As for all women communication is important, but women who have experienced a birth emergency may require additional information and explanations to assist understanding.

A way of assisting women to understand and come to terms with their traumatic birth experience may be by providing postnatal debriefing. Ayers *et al.*[66] identified that 94% of hospitals in the UK provided postnatal services for women who have had a difficult birth. Sixty-five per cent of these services were debriefing services, 13% 'birth afterthoughts' programmes provided by midwives, midwife-counsellors or doctors. The other 22% were psychotherapy (14%) and a service based on individual needs (8%). Five per cent of services were reported to be provided in response to research evidence, the remaining 95% in response to women's perceived needs. It is possible that services have been implemented as a damage limitation measure in response to concerns relating to litigation in obstetrics.[66,67]

Debriefing has been recommended as an intervention, but it is a broad term and has caused confusion in literature and research; also there is controversy with regards to its effectiveness. The need for clarity of terms has been identified by Alexander[68] (*see* Box 13.6). *Making a Difference*[69] recommended that midwives provide 'debriefing'. However, there is little evidence that debriefing interventions are beneficial and some evidence that they may increase the risk of developing PTSD and depression.[70–74] As a result NICE[10] guidelines do not recommend offering a routine single-session formal debriefing to women who have experienced a traumatic birth. However, they do recommend that support be provided for women who wish to talk about their experience and that the effect on the partner should also be considered.

In support of debriefing Lavender and Walkinshaw[75] and Gamble et al.[76] in their randomised studies found that debriefing reduced symptoms of PTSD and PND at three weeks to three months after birth. Also there is evidence that women welcome the opportunity to talk about their birth experience with a supportive health professional, and felt it facilitated their postnatal recovery and adjustment.[77]

Gamble and Creedy[78] subsequently developed a counselling model for postpartum women after a traumatic birth. The results of their study suggest that women are more able to process events surrounding birth at four to six weeks postpartum rather than immediately and that counselling offered too soon may interfere with the woman's ability to process what has happened to her. They identify key elements for counselling support that can be used by midwives, such as showing kindness, listening with encouragement/prompting, clarifying misunderstandings, not justifying or defending care, gently challenging any self-blame, identifying ways to enhance social support etc.

BOX 13.6 Some postnatal interventions intended to reduce PTSD and PND

- **Debriefing** is the most common term used and usually consists of one session within four weeks of a traumatic birth. The session is to encourage the individual to talk about their experience to promote emotional processing and understanding. Psychological debriefing is a type of counselling. Medical debriefing provided by a midwife or doctor may focus more on the medical events and explanations and involve going through their notes.
- **Defusing** is a term used by Alexander[68] to describe midwives giving women the opportunity to talk about their birth during the postnatal period.
- **Listening service** appears to be similar to debriefing and defusing

but the emphasis is on listening. A listening and information service may be one that women can access to discuss unresolved issues in an unlimited time period postpartum.
- **'Birth Afterthoughts'** programmes where women meet with a midwife or midwife counsellor to go over the obstetric events of their birth and express their feelings. These programmes may be similar to listening and information services.
- **Counselling** is an intervention intended to understand the cognitive processes that link the (birth) event with trauma reactions, with the intention of reducing women's distress following a traumatic birth experience. Specialist training would be required for this.

The problems related to ascertaining the effectiveness of debriefing and counselling may be due to inconsistency in the approaches used, and the personal nature of this type of intervention.[77,79] The research tends to focus on the provision of a specific session or sessions rather than providing opportunities for women to talk about their experience and have questions answered when they want. Being able to recount what has happened, to a sympathetic person, has been shown to promote understanding and the regaining of a psychological equilibrium.[78] However, a formal session may result in women revisiting their experience at an inappropriate time and/or being provided with more information than they can cope with.

The opportunity for women to talk about their birth experience and gain the information they need may be provided during routine postnatal care or arranged later when the woman requests it. Women's views of postnatal care have identified that they are frequently not encouraged to ask questions about their birth, how they felt about it and that emotional support was not provided.[77] Therefore, midwives need to ensure they ask women if they have any concerns or questions regarding what happened during the birth of their baby and offer emotional support. Discussion should be led by the woman, to avoid providing more information than she can take in while providing information that will

---

BOX 13.7 Postnatal care following a birth emergency

- Promote parental–baby bonding as appropriate.
- Encourage and facilitate breast feeding as desired by the mother.
- Avoid leaving the woman alone in the initial period.
- Ensure effective postnatal analgesia is provided for women experiencing pain.
- Offer simple explanations and information as desired by the mother and father.
- Offer sympathy and apologies where appropriate; do not justify or defend care given.
- Take into account that women may not want too much information initially, but give information that is needed to facilitate recovery.

- Routine 'debriefing' is not advised and if felt beneficial should be used with caution.
- Provide opportunities and support for women wishing to talk about their experience, encourage use of support from family and friends.
- Consider the effect on the partner and include in postnatal care.
- Refer parents for specialist support (e.g. psychologist or bereavement counsellor) when required.
- Provide information on support so parents can make contact when they feel the need.

assist the mother in helping herself to recover. In this way women will be able to access the information they need and when they want it. The six-week postnatal check may be a more appropriate time for some women to discuss their birth when they have sufficiently recovered from the emergency they experienced. However, only two out of the 10 women in Mapp and Hudson's[1] study understood what had happened to them after their six-week postnatal check with their GP. For this reason Mapp[64] suggests that it may be more appropriate for women who have experienced a birth emergency to have their appointment with a healthcare professional who had an understanding of the events. Partners should also be included in postnatal care and provided with support and information.

If a woman or her partner show any signs of PTSD or PND it is important that they are referred for treatment. Cognitive behaviour therapy has been shown to be effective for PTSD[41] (*see* Box 13.7 for postnatal care following a birth emergency).

Conclusion

Psychological considerations are an essential part of midwifery care when a birth emergency occurs and PTSD and PND are more common in women and their partners following this.[2-4,40] Some women are more at risk of PTSD and PND due to factors other than the birth emergency and these need to be taken into consideration.[25] Information from women and their partners indicates that professionals may focus on the birth emergency and physical care.[1] In doing this the woman and her partner may not be listened to, or informed of what is happening, resulting

in emotions such as anger, fear and loss of control, thus increasing poor psychological outcomes. Working in partnership with the woman and including her partner is necessary to provide the support needed to help the couple cope psychologically following an emergency. The risk of PTSD and PND is increased when women and their partners do not feel supported and have a poor relationship with those providing care. A traumatic birth is 'in the eye of the beholder'[51] and information from parents clearly shows that it is important that caregivers communicate effectively and demonstrate that they care. Feeling the care provided at the time was appropriate and 'the right thing was done' improves the experience of the woman and her partner and facilitates a good psychological outcome.

Following a birth emergency it is important that psychological care is continued to support parent–infant bonding, and assist the couple in coming to terms with what has happened. The couple may initially feel 'shell shocked' so information needs to be provided when they are physically and emotionally able to take it in. Information may need to be repeated with additional explanations, to assist understanding and avoid unresolved issues.

This chapter has considered psychological pathology associated with childbirth and the impact of a traumatic birth. It has identified some risk factors and strategies for reducing the risk of PTSD and PND when a birth emergency occurs. Psychological as well as physical care needs to be included when a birth emergency occurs to improve the outcome for women and their partners. Strategies need to be incorporated in emergency skills training so they can be rehearsed and implemented. Midwives have a key role in providing emotional support and consequently can make a big difference to a woman and her partner's experience, memories and outcomes of childbirth.

References

1 Mapp T, Hudson K. (2005) Feelings and fears during obstetric emergencies – 1. *Br J Midwifery*. **13**(1): 30–5.

2 Wijma K, Ryding EL, Wijma B. (2002) Predicting psychological well-being after emergency caesarean section: a preliminary study. *J Reprod Infant Psychol*. **20**(1): 25–36.

3 Gamble J, Creedy D. (2005) Psychological trauma symptoms of operative birth. *Br J Midwif*. **13**(4): 218–24.

4 White G. (2007) You cope by breaking down in private: fathers and PTSD following childbirth. *Br J Midwif*. **15**(1): 39–45.

5 Soderquist J, Wijma B, Thorbert G, Wijma K. (2009) Risk factors in pregnancy for post-traumatic stress and depression after childbirth. *BJOG*. **116**: 672–80.

6 White T, Matthey S, Boyd K, Barnett B. (2006) Postnatal depression and post-traumatic stress after childbirth: prevalence, course and co-occurrence. *J Reprod Infant Psychol*. **24**(2): 107–20.

7 American Psychiatric Association (APA). (1994) *Diagnostic and Statistical Manual of Mental Disorders*. 4th ed. Washington, DC: American Psychiatric Association.

8 Cox JL, Holden JM, Sagovsky R. (1987) Detection of postnatal depression: development of the 10-item Edinburgh Postnatal Depression Scale. *Br J Psychiatry*. **150**: 782–876.

9 Beck A, Ward C, Mendelsohn M, Mock J, Earbaugh J. (1961) An inventory for measuring depression. *Arch Gen Psychiatry*. **4**: 561–71.

10 National Institute for Clinical Excellence (NICE). (2007) *Antenatal and Postnatal Mental Health: clinical management and service guidance: NICE guideline 45*. London: NICE.

11 Littlewood J, McHugh N. (1997) *Maternal Distress and Postnatal Depression: the myth of the Madonna*. London: Macmillan.

12 Glangeaud-Freudenthal NM-C. (2003) Channi Kumar and the history of the Marce Society. *Arch Womens Ment Health*. **6**(Suppl. 2): S79–82.

13 Shorter E. (1991) *Women's Bodies: a social history of women's encounter with health, ill-health, and medicine*. London: Transaction Publishers.

14 Oakley A. (1993) *Essays on Women Medicine and Health*. Edinburgh: Edinburgh University Press.

15 Radley A. (1994) *Making Sense of Illness: the social psychology of health and disease*. London: Sage Publications.

16 McCourt C. (2009) Social support and childbirth. In: Squire C, editor. *The Social Context of Birth*. 2nd ed. Oxford: Radcliffe Medical Press.

17 Schneider Z. (2002) An Australian study of women's experiences of their first pregnancy. *Midwifery*. **18**: 238–49.

18 Pitt B. (1968) Atypical depression following childbirth. *Br J Psychiatry*. **114**: 1325–35.

19 Murray L, Cooper PJ. (1997) *Postpartum Depression and Child Development*. London: The Guildford Press.

20 Brockington IF, Cernick KF, Schofield EM, Downing AR, Francis AF, Keelan C. (1981) Puerperal psychosis: phenomena and diagnosis. *Arch Gen Psychiatry*. **38**: 829–33.

21 Beck CT, Driscoll JD. (2006) *Postpartum Mood and Anxiety Disorders: a clinician's guide*. London: Jones and Bartlett.

22 Wijma K. (2006) Post-traumatic stress disorder and childbirth. In: Keane V, Marsh M, Seneviratne G, editors. *Psychiatric Disorders and Pregnancy*. London: Taylor & Francis.

23 American Psychiatric Association (APA). (1987) *Diagnostic and Statistical Manual of Mental Disorders*. 3rd ed., revised. Washington: American Psychiatric Association.

24 Leeds L, Hargreaves I. (2008) The psychological consequences of childbirth. *J Reprod Infant Psychol*. **26**(2): 108–22.

25 Ryding EL, Wijma K, Wijma B. (2000) Emergency cesarean section: 25 women's experiences. *J Reprod Infant Psychol.* **18**(1): 33–9.

26 Menage J. (1993) Post traumatic stress disorder in women who have undergone obstetric and/or gynaecological procedures. *J Reprod Infant Psychol.* **11**(4): 221–8.

27 Bowman ML. (1999) Individual differences in posttraumatic distress: problems with the DSM-IV model. *Can J Psychiatry.* **44**: 21–33.

28 Lewis G, editor. (2007) *Confidential Enquiry into Maternal and Child Health (CEMACH). Saving Mothers' Lives: reviewing maternal deaths to make motherhood safer – 2003–2005. The Seventh Report on Confidential Enquiries into Maternal Deaths in the United Kingdom.* London: CEMACH.

29 Zar M, Wijma K, Wijma B. (2002) Relation between anxiety disorders and fear of childbirth during late pregnancy. *Clin Psychol Psychother.* **9**: 122–30.

30 Fones C. (1996) Post-traumatic stress disorder occurring after painful childbirth. *J Nerv Ment Dis.* **18**: 195–6.

31 Department of Health (DH). (1993) *Changing Childbirth, Part 1: Report of the Expert Maternity Group.* London: HMSO.

32 Department of Health (DH). (2004) *National Service Framework for Children, Young People and Maternity Services.* London: HMSO.

33 Department of Health (DH). (2007) *Maternity Matters: choice, access and continuity of care in a safe service.* London: HMSO.

34 Beech B, Robinson J. (1985) Nightmares following childbirth. *Br J Psychiatry.* **147**: 586.

35 Kitzinger S. (2004) Flashbacks, nightmares and panic attacks after birth. *Br J Midwif.* **12**(1): 12.

36 Kitzinger S. (2005) *The Politics of Birth.* London: Elsevier.

37 Green JM, Coupland VA, Kitzinger JV. (1998) *Great Expectations: a prospective study of women's expectations and experiences of childbirth.* 2nd ed. Hale

Cheshire: Books for Midwives Press.

38 Lyons S. (1998) Post-traumatic stress disorder following childbirth: causes, prevention and treatment. In: Clement S, editor. *Psychological Perspectives on Pregnancy and Childbirth.* London: Churchill Livingstone.

39 Soderquist J, Wijma B, Wijma K. (2006) The longitudinal course of post-traumatic stress after childbirth. *J Psychsom Obstet Gynaecol.* **27**(2): 113–19.

40 Creedy D, Shochet I, Horsfall J. (2000) Childbirth and the development of acute trauma symptoms: incidence and contributing factors. *Birth.* **27**(2): 104–11.

41 Ayers S, McKenzie-McHarg K, Eagle A. (2007) Cognitive behaviour therapy for postnatal post-traumatic stress disorder: case studies. *J Psychosom Obstet Gynaecol.* **28**(3): 177–84.

42 Ayers S, Wright DB, Wells N. (2007) Symptoms of post-traumatic stress disorder in couples after birth: association with the couple's relationship and parent-baby bond. *J Reprod Infant Psychol.* **25**(1): 40–50.

43 Longworth H. (2006) Should fathers be in the labour room? Yes, for support not intervention. *Br J Midwif.* **14**(5): 288.

44 Parfitt YM, Ayers S. (2009) The effect of post-natal symptoms of post-traumatic stress and depression on the couple's relationship and parent-baby bond. *J Reprod Infant Psychol.* **27**(2): 127–42.

45 Skari H, Skreden M, Malt UF, Dalholt M, Ostensen AB, Egeland T, Emblem R. (2002) Comparative levels of psychological distress, stress symptoms, depression and anxiety after childbirth: a prospective population-based study of mothers and fathers. *BJOG.* **109**: 1154–63.

46 Breslau N, Davis G, Andreski P, Peterson E, Schultz LR. (1997) Sex differences in posttraumatic stress disorder. *Arch Womens Ment Health.* **9**: 1044–8.

47 O'Hara MW, Swain AM. (1996) Rates and risk of postpartum depression: a meta-analysis. *Int Rev Psychiatry.* **8**: 37–54.

48 Ballard CG, Stanly AK, Brockington IF. (1995) Posttraumatic stress disorder after childbirth. *Br J Psychiatry.* **166**: 525–8.

49 Czarnocka J, Slade P. (2000) Prevalence and predictors of post-traumatic stress symptoms following childbirth. *Br J Clin Psychol.* **39**: 25–51.

50 Joseph S, Bailham D. (2004) Traumatic childbirth: what we know and what we can do. *Midwives.* **7**(6): 258–61.

51 Beck CT. (2004) Birth trauma in the eye of the beholder. *Nurs Res.* **53**(1): 28–35.

52 Trowell J. (1982) Possible effects of emergency caesarean section: a research study of the mother/child relationship. *Early Hum Dev.* **7**: 41–51.

53 Calam RM, Lambrenos K, Cox AD, Weindling AM. (1999) Maternal appraisal of information given around the time of preterm delivery. *J Reprod Infant Psychol.* **17**(3): 267–80.

54 Ayers S. (2007) Thoughts and emotions during traumatic birth: a qualitative study. *Birth.* **34**(3): 253–63.

55 Mitchell D, Chapman P. (2002) *Part of the Team or Warming the Bench?* Nelson, NZ: Nelson Marlborough Institute of Technology, Nelson Marlborough District Health Board.

56 National Collaborating Centre for Women's and Children's Health. (2007) *Intrapartum Care: care of healthy women and their babies during childbirth.* London: RCOG Press.

57 Zauderer C, Galea E. (2010) Breastfeeding and depression: empowering the new mother. *Br J Midwif.* **18**(2): 88–91.

58 Erlandsson K, Dsilna A, Fagerberg I, Christensson K. (2007) Skin-to-skin care with the father after cesarean birth and its effect on newborn crying and prefeeding behavior. *Birth.* **34**(2): 105–13.

59 Obeidat HM, Bond EA, Callister LC. (2009) The parental experience of having an infant in the newborn intensive care unit. *J Perinat Educ.* **18**(3): 23–9.

60 Sargent AN. (2009) Predictors of needs in mothers with infants in the neonatal intensive care unit. *J Reprod Infant Psychol.* **27**(2): 195–205.

61 Crathern L. (2009) Dads matter too: a review of the literature focusing on the experiences of fathers of preterm infants. *MIDIRS Midwifery Digest.* **19**(2): 159–67.

62 Brockington IF. (2004) Diagnosis and management of post-partum disorders: a review. *World Psychiatry.* **3**: 89–95.

63 Wenzel A, Haugen EN, Jackson LC, Brendle JR. (2005) Anxiety symptoms and disorders at eight weeks postpartum. *J Anxiety Disord.* **19**: 295–311.

64 Mapp T. (2005) Feelings and fears post obstetric emergencies – 2. *Br J Midwif.* **13**(1): 36–40.

65 National Institute for Clinical Excellence (NICE). (2006) *Routine Postnatal Care of Women and their Babies: NICE guideline 37.* London: NICE.

66 Ayers S, Claypool J, Eagle A. (2006) What happens after a difficult birth? Postnatal debriefing services. *Br J Midwif.* **14**(3): 157–61.

67 Symon A. (1997) Improving communication: apologies and explanations. *Br J Midwif.* **5**(10): 594–6.

68 Alexander J. (1998) Confusing debriefing and defusing postnatally: the need for clarity of terms, purpose and value. *Midwifery.* **14**: 122–4.

69 Department of Health (DH). (1999) *Making a Difference.* London: HMSO.

70 Gamble J, Creedy D, Webster J, Moyle W. (2002) A review of the literature on debriefing or non-directive counselling to prevent postpartum emotional distress. *Midwifery.* **18**: 72–9.

71 Kershaw K, Jolly J, Bhabra K, Ford J. (2005) Randomised controlled trial of community debriefing following operative delivery. *Br J Obstet Gynaecol.* **112**: 1504–9.

72 Priest SR, Henderson J, Evans SF, Hagan R. (2003) Stress debriefing after childbirth: a randomised controlled trial. *Med J Aust.* **178**: 542–5.

73 Rose S, Bisson J, Churchill R, Wessely S. (2002) Psychological debriefing for preventing post-traumatic stress disorder. *Cochrane Database Syst Rev.* **2**: CD000560.

74 Small R, Lumley J, Donohue L, Potter A, Waldenstrom U. (2000) Randomised controlled trial of midwife led debriefing to reduce maternal depression after operative birth. *BMJ.* **321**: 1043–7.

75 Lavender T, Walkinshaw SA. (1998)

Can midwives reduce postpartum psychological morbidity? A randomised controlled trial. *Birth*. 25: 215–19.

76 Gamble J, Creedy D, Moyle W, Webster J, McAllister M, Dickson P. (2005) Effectiveness of a counselling intervention after a traumatic childbirth: a randomised controlled trial. *Birth*. 32: 11–19.

77 Gamble J, Creedy D. (2004) Content and process of postpartum counselling after a distressing birth experience: a review. *Birth*. 31(3): 213–18.

78 Gamble J, Creedy D. (2009) A counselling model for postpartum women after distressing birth experiences. *Midwifery*. 25: e21–e30.

79 Kitzinger C, Kitzinger S. (2007) Birth trauma: talking with women and the value of conversation analysis. *Br J Midwifery*. 15(5): 256–64.

Index